ORTHOPEDIC CLINICS OF NORTH AMERICA

www.orthopedic.theclinics.com

Orthobiologics

July 2017 • Volume 48 • Number 3

Editor-in-Chief

FREDERICK M. AZAR

Editorial Board

JAMES H. CALANDRUCCIO
BENJAMIN J. GREAR
BENJAMIN M. MAUCK
JEFFREY R. SAWYER
PATRICK C. TOY
JOHN C. WEINLEIN

ELSEVIER

1600 John F. Kennedy Boulevard • Suite 1800 • Philadelphia, Pennsylvania, 19103-2899.

http://www.orthopedic.theclinics.com

ORTHOPEDIC CLINICS OF NORTH AMERICA Volume 48, Number 3
July 2017 ISSN 0030-5898, ISBN-13: 978-0-323-53142-9

Editor: Lauren Boyle
Developmental Editor: Kristen Helm

Photocopying

Single photocopies of single articles may be made for personal use as allowed by national copyright laws. Permission of the Publisher and payment of a fee is required for all other photocopying, including multiple or systematic copying, copying for advertising or promotional purposes, resale, and all forms of document delivery. Special rates are available for educational institutions that wish to make photocopies for non-profit educational classroom use. For information on how to seek permission visit www.elsevier.com/permissions or call: (+44) 1865 843830 (UK)/(+1) 215 239 3804 (USA).

Derivative Works

Subscribers may reproduce tables of contents or prepare lists of articles including abstracts for internal circulation within their institutions. Permission of the Publisher is required for resale or distribution outside the institution. Permission of the Publisher is required for all other derivative works, including compilations and translations (please consult www.elsevier.com/permissions).

Electronic Storage or Usage

Permission of the Publisher is required to store or use electronically any material contained in this periodical, including any article or part of an article (please consult www.elsevier.com/permissions). Except as outlined above, no part of this publication may be reproduced, stored in a retrieval system or transmitted in any form or by any means, electronic, mechanical, photocopying, recording or otherwise, without prior written permission of the Publisher.

Notice

No responsibility is assumed by the Publisher for any injury and/or damage to persons or property as a matter of products liability, negligence or otherwise, or from any use or operation of any methods, products, instructions or ideas contained in the material herein. Because of rapid advances in the medical sciences, in particular, independent verification of diagnoses and drug dosages should be made.

Although all advertising material is expected to conform to ethical (medical) standards, inclusion in this publication does not constitute a guarantee or endorsement of the quality or value of such product or of the claims made of it by its manufacturer.

Orthopedic Clinics of North America (ISSN 0030-5898) is published quarterly by Elsevier Inc., 360 Park Avenue South, New York, NY 10010-1710. Months of issue are January, April, July, and October. Business and Editorial Offices: 1600 John F. Kennedy Blvd., Suite 1800, Philadelphia, PA 19103-2899. Customer Service Office: 3251 Riverport Lane, Maryland Heights, MO 63043. Periodicals postage paid at New York, NY and additional mailing offices. Subscription prices are $319.00 per year for (US individuals), $686.00 per year for (US institutions), $376.00 per year (Canadian individuals), $837.00 per year (Canadian institutions), $464.00 per year (international individuals), $837.00 per year (international institutions), $100.00 per year (US students), $220.00 per year (Canadian and international students). Foreign air speed delivery is included in all *Clinics* subscription prices. All prices are subject to change without notice. **POSTMASTER:** Send change of address to *Orthopedic Clinics of North America*, **Elsevier Health Sciences Division, Subscription Customer Service, 3251 Riverport Lane, Maryland Heights, MO 63043. Customer Service (orders, claims, online, change of address): Elsevier Health Sciences Division, Subscription Customer Service, 3251 Riverport Lane, Maryland Heights, MO 63043. Tel: 1-800-654-2452 (U.S. and Canada); 314-447-8871 (outside U.S. and Canada). Fax: 314-447-8029. E-mail:** journalscustomerservice-usa@elsevier.com **(for print support);** journalsonlinesupport-usa@elsevier.com **(for online support).**

Reprints. For copies of 100 or more, of articles in this publication, please contact the Commercial Reprints Department, Elsevier Inc., 360 Park Avenue South, New York, NY 10010-1710. Tel.: 212-633-3874; Fax: 212-633-3820; E-mail: reprints@elsevier.com.

Orthopedic Clinics of North America is covered in MEDLINE/PubMed (Index Medicus), Cinahl, Excerpta Medica, and Cumulative Index to Nursing and Allied Health Literature.

PROGRAM OBJECTIVE

Orthopedic Clinics of North America offers clinical review articles on the most cutting-edge technologies and techniques in the field, including adult reconstruction, the upper extremity, pediatrics, trauma, oncology, and sports medicine.

TARGET AUDIENCE

Practicing orthopedic surgeons, orthopedic residents, and other healthcare professionals who specialize in orthopedic technologies and techniques for adult reconstruction, the upper extremity, pediatrics, trauma, oncology, and sports medicine.

LEARNING OBJECTIVES

Upon completion of this activity, participants will be able to:
1. Review the role of orthobiologics in pediatric orthopedics and sports medicine.
2. Discuss tissue engineering in joint arthroplasty and fracture treatment.
3. Recognize the use of orthobiologics in treatment of problems of the extremities.

ACCREDITATION

The Elsevier Office of Continuing Medical Education (EOCME) is accredited by the Accreditation Council for Continuing Medical Education (ACCME) to provide continuing medical education for physicians.

The EOCME designates this enduring material for a maximum of 15 *AMA PRA Category 1 Credit*(s)™. Physicians should claim only the credit commensurate with the extent of their participation in the activity.

All other healthcare professionals requesting continuing education credit for this enduring material will be issued a certificate of participation.

DISCLOSURE OF CONFLICTS OF INTEREST

The EOCME assesses conflict of interest with its instructors, faculty, planners, and other individuals who are in a position to control the content of CME activities. All relevant conflicts of interest that are identified are thoroughly vetted by EOCME for fair balance, scientific objectivity, and patient care recommendations. EOCME is committed to providing its learners with CME activities that promote improvements or quality in healthcare and not a specific proprietary business or a commercial interest.

The planning committee, staff, authors and editors listed below have identified no financial relationships or relationships to products or devices they or their spouse/life partner have with commercial interest related to the content of this CME activity:

Frederick M. Azar, MD; Eric A. Barcak, DO; Michael J. Beebe, MD; Lauren Boyle; Christopher C. Bray, MD; James H. Calandruccio, MD; Peter N. Chalmers, MD; John Chao, MD; Brian J. Cole, MD, MBA; Craig J. Della Valle, MD; Mouhanad M. El-Othmani, MD; Anjali Fortna; Rachel M. Frank, MD; Todd J. Frush, MD; Kristen Helm; Gerard Insley, PhD; James F. Mooney III, MD; Robert F. Murphy, MD; Andrew Pao, MD; Darren Plummer, MD, MBA; Khaled J. Saleh, MD, MSc, FRCS(C), MHCM, CPE; Zeina M. Saleh, MD; Patrick C. Schottel, MD; David D. Spence, MD; Murphy M. Steiner, MD; Jeyanthi Surendrakumar; Brandon A. Taylor, MD; Clark M. Walker, MD; Stephen J. Warner, MD, PhD; Katie Widmeier; Amy Williams; Jane C. Yeoh, MD, FRCSC; Hussein A. Zeineddine, MD.

The planning committee, staff, authors and editors listed below have identified financial relationships or relationships to products or devices they or their spouse/life partner have with commercial interest related to the content of this CME activity:

Thomas A. Russell, MD is on the speakers' bureau for, a consultant/advisor for, and receives royalties/patents from Zimmer Biomet, and receives royalties/patents from Smith and Nephew.

UNAPPROVED/OFF-LABEL USE DISCLOSURE

The EOCME requires CME faculty to disclose to the participants:
1. When products or procedures being discussed are off-label, unlabelled, experimental, and/or investigational (not US Food and Drug Administration [FDA] approved); and
2. Any limitations on the information presented, such as data that are preliminary or that represent ongoing research, interim analyses, and/or unsupported opinions. Faculty may discuss information about pharmaceutical agents that is outside of FDA-approved labelling. This information is intended solely for CME and is not intended to promote off-label use of these medications. If you have any questions, contact the medical affairs department of the manufacturer for the most recent prescribing information.

TO ENROLL

To enroll in the *Orthopedic Clinics of North America* Continuing Medical Education program, call customer service at 1-800-654-2452 or sign up online at http://www.theclinics.com/home/cme. The CME program is available to subscribers for an additional annual fee of USD 215.

METHOD OF PARTICIPATION

In order to claim credit, participants must complete the following:
1. Complete enrolment as indicated above.
2. Read the activity.

3. Complete the CME Test and Evaluation. Participants must achieve a score of 70% on the test. All CME Tests and Evaluations must be completed online.

CME INQUIRIES/SPECIAL NEEDS

For all CME inquiries or special needs, please contact elsevierCME@elsevier.com.

EDITORIAL BOARD

FREDERICK M. AZAR, MD – EDITOR-IN-CHIEF
Professor, Department of Orthopaedic Surgery & Biomedical Engineering,
University of Tennessee-Campbell Clinic; Chief-of-Staff, Campbell Clinic, Inc,
Memphis, Tennessee

PATRICK C. TOY, MD – ADULT RECONSTRUCTION
Assistant Professor, Department of Orthopaedic Surgery & Biomedical
Engineering, University of Tennessee-Campbell Clinic, Memphis, Tennessee

JOHN C. WEINLEIN, MD – TRAUMA
Assistant Professor, University of Tennessee-Campbell Clinic, Elvis Presley
Memorial Trauma Center, Regional One Health, Memphis, Tennessee

JEFFREY R. SAWYER, MD – PEDIATRICS
Professor of Orthopaedic Surgery; Director, Pediatric Orthopaedic Fellowship,
University of Tennessee-Campbell Clinic, Memphis, Tennessee

BENJAMIN M. MAUCK, MD – UPPER EXTREMITY
Hand and Upper Extremity Surgery, Campbell Clinic; Clinical Instructor,
Department of Orthopedic Surgery, University of Tennessee Health Science
Center, Memphis, Tennessee

JAMES H. CALANDRUCCIO, MD – UPPER EXTREMITY
Assistant Professor, Department of Orthopaedic Surgery and Biomedical
Engineering, University of Tennessee-Campbell Clinic; Staff Physician, Campbell
Clinic, Inc, Memphis, Tennessee

BENJAMIN J. GREAR, MD – FOOT AND ANKLE
Instructor, Department of Orthopaedic Surgery and Biomedical Engineering,
University of Tennessee-Campbell Clinic; Staff Physician, Campbell Clinic, Inc,
Memphis, Tennessee

CONTRIBUTORS

AUTHORS

ERIC A. BARCAK, DO
Orthopedic Surgery Trauma Fellow, University of Tennessee–Campbell Clinic, Memphis, Tennessee

MICHAEL J. BEEBE, MD
Assistant Professor of Orthopedic Surgery, University of Tennessee–Campbell Clinic, Memphis, Tennessee

CHRISTOPHER C. BRAY, MD
Pediatric Orthopaedic Surgery and Adolescent Sports Medicine, Assistant Program Director, Department of Orthopaedic Surgery, Steadman Hawkins Clinic of the Carolinas, Greenville Health System, Assistant Professor, University of South Carolina School of Medicine-Greenville, Greenville, South Carolina

JAMES H. CALANDRUCCIO, MD
Associate Professor, Department of Orthopaedic Surgery and Biomedical Engineering, University of Tennessee–Campbell Clinic, Memphis, Tennessee

PETER N. CHALMERS, MD
Department of Orthopaedic Surgery, Rush University Medical Center, Chicago, Illinois

JOHN CHAO, MD
Clinical Faculty, Atlanta Medical Center, Peachtree Orthopaedic Clinic, Atlanta, Georgia

BRIAN J. COLE, MD, MBA
Professor and Associate Chairman, Department of Orthopaedic Surgery, Rush University Medical Center, Chicago, Illinois

CRAIG J. DELLA VALLE, MD
Professor and Chief of Adult Reconstructive Surgery, Department of Orthopaedic Surgery, Rush University Medical Center, Chicago, Illinois

MOUHANAD M. EL-OTHMANI, MD
Clinical Research Assistant, Department of Orthopaedics and Sports Medicine, Musculoskeletal Institute of Excellence, Detroit Medical Center, University Health Center, Detroit, Michigan

RACHEL M. FRANK, MD
Department of Orthopaedic Surgery, Rush University Medical Center, Chicago, Illinois

TODD J. FRUSH, MD
Associate Program Director, Department of Orthopaedics and Sports Medicine, Detroit Medical Center, University Health Center, Detroit, Michigan

GERARD INSLEY, PhD
Chief Scientific Officer, Celgen Tek, Shannon, Co. Clare, Ireland

JAMES F. MOONEY III, MD
Professor, Department of Orthopaedics, Medical University of South Carolina, Charleston, South Carolina

ROBERT F. MURPHY, MD
Assistant Professor, Department of Orthopaedics, Medical University of South Carolina, Charleston, South Carolina

ANDREW PAO, MD
Atlanta Medical Center, Atlanta, Georgia

DARREN R. PLUMMER, MD, MBA
Department of Orthopaedic Surgery, Rush University Medical Center, Chicago, Illinois

THOMAS A. RUSSELL, MD
Professor (Ret.), Department of Orthopedic Surgery, Campbell Clinic, University of Tennessee Center for the Health Sciences, University of Tennessee, Memphis, Tennessee

KHALED J. SALEH, MD, MSc, FRCS(C), MHCM, CPE
Executive-In-Chief, Department of Orthopaedics and Sports Medicine, Detroit Medical Center, University Health Center, Detroit, Michigan

ZEINA M. SALEH, MD
Clinical Scholar, Department of Surgery, American University of Beirut Medical Center, Beirut, Lebanon

PATRICK C. SCHOTTEL, MD
Assistant Professor, Department of
Orthopaedic Surgery and Rehabilitation,
University of Vermont College of Medicine,
Burlington, Vermont

DAVID D. SPENCE, MD
Assistant Professor, Department of
Orthopaedic Surgery, University of
Tennessee–Campbell Clinic, Memphis,
Tennessee

MURPHY M. STEINER, MD
Hand Surgery Fellow, Department of
Orthopaedic Surgery and Biomedical
Engineering, University of Tennessee–
Campbell Clinic, Memphis, Tennessee

BRANDON A. TAYLOR, MD
Fellow, Campbell Clinic Foot & Ankle
Department, Germantown, Tennessee

CLARK M. WALKER, MD
Department of Orthopaedic Surgery,
Greenville Health System, Greenville,
South Carolina

STEPHEN J. WARNER, MD, PhD
Orthopaedic Trauma Fellow, Department of
Orthopaedic Surgery, University of Texas
Health Science Center at Houston, Houston,
Texas

JANE C. YEOH, MD, FRCSC
Fellow, Campbell Clinic Foot & Ankle
Department, Germantown, Tennessee

HUSSEIN A. ZEINEDDINE, MD
Postdoctoral Scholar, Department of Surgery,
University of Chicago Medical Center,
Chicago, Illinois

CONTENTS

Adult Reconstruction
Patrick C. Toy

This study compared patients who failed a cartilage restoration procedure and underwent ipsilateral knee arthroplasty with matched control subjects undergoing knee arthroplasty without prior cartilage restoration. Although patients with a failed cartilage procedure derived benefit from knee arthroplasty, their magnitude of improvement and final outcomes scores were lower than the matched control subjects. In this cohort, the cartilage patients also experienced little to no benefit from cartilage restoration, suggesting that unmeasured shared patient characteristics may play a role. This information can be used to counsel this difficult patient population on expected outcomes following arthroplasty procedures. Further research identifying characteristics of responders to treatment remains critical to refine clinical decision-making for this difficult patient group.

Research in tissue engineering has undoubtedly achieved significant milestones in recent years. Although it is being applied in several disciplines, tissue engineering's application is particularly advanced in orthopedic surgery and in degenerative joint diseases. The literature is full of remarkable findings and trials using tissue engineering in articular cartilage disease. With the vast and expanding knowledge, and with the variety of techniques available at hand, the authors aimed to review the current concepts and advances in the use of cell sources in articular cartilage tissue engineering.

Trauma
John C. Weinlein

This article focuses on the understanding of the biochemistry and surgical application of bone substitute materials (BSMs) and particularly the newer calcium phosphate materials that can form a structural orthobiologic matrix within the metaphyseal components of the periarticular bone. Six characteristics of BSMs are detailed that can be used as a guide for the proper selection and application of the optimal BSM type for periarticular fracture repair. These 6 characteristics of BSMs are divided into 2 pillars. One pillar details the 3 biochemical features of BSMs and the other pillar details the 3 surgical application properties.

Approximately 10 years ago bone morphogenic protein (BMP) was seen as a miraculous adjuvant to assist with bone growth. However, in the face of an increasing number of complications and a lack of understanding its long-term effects, it is unclear what role BMP has in the current treatment of orthopedic trauma patients. This article reviews the current recommendations, trends, and associated complications of BMP use in fracture care.

Bone marrow aspirate grafting entails mesenchymal stem cell-containing bone marrow harvesting and injection into a fracture site to promote bone formation. Although the use of bone marrow aspirate in orthopedic trauma is not widespread, an increasing number of studies are reporting clinical success. Advantages of using bone marrow aspirate are that it is readily obtainable, has low harvest morbidity, and can be easily and quickly injected. However, no universally accepted role for its use exists. Future studies directly comparing bone marrow aspirate with conventional techniques are needed to define its role in the treatment of orthopedic trauma patients.

Pediatrics
Jeffrey R. Sawyer

Orthobiologics are biologic devices or products used in orthopedic surgery to augment or enhance bone formation. The use of orthobiologics in pediatric orthopedics is less frequent than in other orthopedic subspecialties, mainly due to the naturally abundant healing potential and bone formation in children compared with adults. However, orthobiologics are used in certain situations in pediatric orthopedics, particularly in spine and foot surgery. Other uses have been reported in conjunction with specific procedures involving the tibia and pelvis. The use of bioabsorable implants to stabilize children's fractures is an emerging concept but has limited supporting data.

Orthobiologics are biological substances that allow injured muscles, tendons, ligaments, and bone to heal more quickly. They are found naturally in the body; at higher concentrations they can aid in the healing process. These substances include autograft bone, allograft bone, demineralized bone matrix, bone morphogenic proteins, growth factors, stem cells, plasma-rich protein, and ceramic grafts. Their use in sports medicine has exploded in efforts to increase graft incorporation, stimulate healing, and get athletes back to sport with problems including anterior cruciate ligament ruptures, tendon ruptures, cartilage injuries, and fractures. This article reviews orthobiologics and their applications in pediatric sports medicine.

Upper Extremity
Benjamin M. Mauck and James H. Calandruccio

Orthobiologics are not used as frequently in the hand and wrist as in other sites. The most frequently reported is the use of bone morphogenetic protein for the treatment of Kienböck disease. Animal studies have described improved tendon healing with the use of platelet-rich plasma (PRP), but no clinical studies have confirmed these results. PRP has been reported to produce improvements in the outcomes of distal radial fractures and osteoarthritis of the trapeziometacarpal in small numbers of patients. The use of orthobiologics in the hand and wrist are promising, but clinical trials are necessary to establish efficacy and safety.

Lateral epicondylitis (tennis elbow) is a frequent cause of elbow pain; most patients (80%–90%) are successfully treated with standard nonoperative methods (rest, nonsteroidal anti-inflammatory drugs, bracing, and physical therapy). Autologous blood injections and platelet-rich plasma injections are the two most frequently used orthobiologic techniques in the treatment of lateral epicondylitis. Studies of the effectiveness of autologous blood injections and platelet-rich plasma report varying outcomes, some citing significant clinical relief and others reporting no beneficial effect. More research is needed to determine how to best use orthobiologics in the treatment of lateral epicondylitis.

Foot and Ankle
Benjamin J. Grear

In the surgical treatment of foot and ankle abnormality, many problems require bone grafting for successful osseous union. Nonunion, reconstruction, and arthrodesis procedures pose specific challenges due to bony defects secondary to trauma, malunions, or previous surgery. Nonunion in foot and ankle arthrodesis is a significant risk and is well documented in recent literature. This article is a review of the recent literature regarding the use of bone graft and orthobiologics in foot and ankle surgery.

Symptomatic osteochondral lesions of the talus remain a challenging problem due to inability for cartilage lesions to heal. Numerous treatment options exist, including nonoperative management, marrow stimulating techniques, and autograft-allograft. Arthroscopic marrow stimulation forms fibrocartilage that has been shown to be biomechanically weaker than hyaline cartilage. Restorative tissue transplantation options are being used more for larger and cystic lesions. Newer biologics and particulated juvenile cartilage are currently under investigation for possible clinical efficacy. This article provides an evidenced-based summary of available literature on the use of biologics for treatment of osteochondral lesions of the talus.

ORTHOBIOLOGICS

FORTHCOMING ISSUES

October 2017
Perioperative Pain Management
Clayton C. Bettin, James H. Calandruccio,
Benjamin J. Grear, Benjamin M. Mauck,
Jeffrey R. Sawyer, Patrick C. Toy, and
John C. Weinlein, *Editors*

January 2018
Outpatient Surgery
Michael J. Beebe, Clayton C. Bettin,
James H. Calandruccio, Benjamin J. Grear,
Benjamin M. Mauck, William M. Mihalko,
Jeffrey R. Sawyer, Thomas Q. Throckmorton,
Patrick C. Toy, and John C. Weinlein, *Editors*

April 2018
Evidence-Based Medicine
Michael J. Beebe, Clayton C. Bettin,
James H. Calandruccio, Benjamin J. Grear,
Benjamin M. Mauck, William M. Mihalko,
Jeffrey R. Sawyer, Thomas Q. Throckmorton,
Patrick C. Toy, and John C. Weinlein, *Editors*

RECENT ISSUES

April 2017
Infection
James H. Calandruccio, Benjamin J. Grear,
Benjamin M. Mauck, Jeffrey R. Sawyer,
Patrick C. Toy, and John C. Weinlein, *Editors*

January 2017
Controversies in Fracture Care
James H. Calandruccio, Benjamin J. Grear,
Benjamin M. Mauck, Jeffrey R. Sawyer,
Patrick C. Toy, and John C. Weinlein, *Editors*

October 2016
Sports-Related Injuries
James H. Calandruccio, Benjamin J. Grear,
Benjamin M. Mauck, Jeffrey R. Sawyer,
Patrick C. Toy, and John C. Weinlein, *Editors*

ISSUES OF RELATED INTEREST

Physical Medicine and Rehabilitation Clinics of North America
November 2016 (Vol. 27, No. 4)
Regenerative Medicine
Santos F. Martinez, *Editor*
Available at: http://www.pmr.theclinics.com/

Foot and Ankle Clinics of North America, December 2016 (Vol. 21, No. 4)
Bone Grafts, Bone Graft Substitutes, and Biologics in Foot and Ankle Surgery
Sheldon Lin, *Editor*
Available at: http://www.foot.theclinics.com/

PREFACE

Orthobiologics

This issue of *Orthopedic Clinics of North America* is especially interesting and exciting, with up-to-date information on some of the newest tools available to orthopedists—orthobiologics. From older patients with total joint arthroplasty to children and adolescents with sports injuries, orthobiologics can enhance healing and, in some situations, induce regeneration of injured tissues.

The effect of cartilage restoration techniques on subsequent total knee arthroplasty is explored by Drs Frank, Della Valle, Plummer, Chalmers, and Cole, while Drs Zeineddine, Frush, Z. Saleh, El-Othmani, and K. Saleh review the current concepts and advances in the use of tissue engineering in the treatment of degenerative joint disorders that often require total joint arthroplasty.

The use of orthobiologics in trauma patients is thoroughly reviewed in three related articles on bone substitutes, bone morphogenetic protein (BMP), and bone marrow aspirate. Drs Russell and Insley describe the biochemistry and surgical application of bone substitute material, particularly the newer calcium phosphate materials, and present a guide for proper selection and application. Drs Barcak and Beebe review the current recommendations, trends, and complications of the use of BMP in orthopedic trauma, and Drs Schottel and Warner report the increased use of bone marrow aspirate in trauma situations.

A number of orthobiologic materials have been used in pediatric patients, including autograft and allograft bone, demineralized bone matrix, BMP, growth factors, stem cells, plasma-rich protein (PRP), and ceramic grafts. Drs Murphy and Mooney give a concise overview of the use of these materials in pediatric orthopedic surgery, especially of the spine, foot, tibia, and pelvis, as well as bioabsorbable implants for fracture fixation. Drs Bray, Walker, and Spence narrow the focus to the use of orthobiologics in pediatric sports medicine injuries, such as tendon, ligament, and cartilage injuries.

Although orthobiologics are used less frequently in the upper extremity than in other anatomical sites, Dr Steiner and Calandruccio review their use for treatment of several hand and wrist disorders as well as the use of PRP and autologous blood injections for the treatment of lateral epicondylitis.

Drs Yeoh and Taylor, and Chao and Pao describe and discuss orthobiologics use in foot and ankle disorders and surgeries, including reconstructive bony procedures and treatment of osteochondral lesions of the talus.

Overall, this issue gives you information to help choose and use these promising adjuncts to standard orthopedic techniques. We hope you will find the articles helpful in providing the best care possible to your patients.

Frederick M. Azar, MD
Department of Orthopaedic Surgery
and Biomedical Engineering
University of Tennessee–Campbell Clinic
1211 Union Avenue, Suite 510
Memphis, TN 38104, USA

E-mail address:
fazar@campbellclinic.com

Orthop Clin N Am 48 (2017) xiii
http://dx.doi.org/10.1016/j.ocl.2017.03.012
0030-5898/17/© 2017 Published by Elsevier Inc.

Adult Reconstruction

Does Prior Cartilage Restoration Impact Outcomes Following Knee Arthroplasty?

Rachel M. Frank, MD*, Craig J. Della Valle, MD,
Darren R. Plummer, MD, MBA, Peter N. Chalmers, MD,
Brian J. Cole, MD, MBA

KEYWORDS

- Cartilage restoration • Meniscus transplantation • Knee joint preservation • Arthroplasty

---

KEY POINTS

- When compared with matched control subjects, patients undergoing arthroplasty after prior cartilage/meniscal restoration have significantly less pain relief, lower functional outcomes, and less improvement following partial or total knee arthroplasty.
- Patients undergoing arthroplasty after prior cartilage/meniscal restoration have significantly less severe arthritic findings on radiographs as measured by the Kellegren and Lawrence grade compared with matched control subjects.
- In this study, patients who underwent arthroplasty after failed prior cartilage/meniscal restoration did not experience symptom relief after cartilage/meniscal restoration, which is atypical of the typical patient undergoing cartilage/meniscal restoration.

INTRODUCTION

Injuries to the articular cartilage of the knee are seen in up to 63% of arthroscopies.[1,2] Articular cartilage defects do not reliably heal and can lead to degenerative joint disease,[3–5] ultimately resulting in significant pain and disability.[6–10] The optimal treatment strategy for these defects, one that provides the highest likelihood of a painless return to activity, remains unknown.[6–10] In particular, young, active patients with symptomatic articular cartilage defects are challenging, because arthroplasty may lead to wear-related complications and a need for multiple revisions over an individual's lifetime[11] and hence articular cartilage and meniscal restoration procedures are being performed with increasing frequency.[12–14]

Techniques including autologous chondrocyte implantation or variations thereof (**Fig. 1**), osteochondral autograft transfer, osteochondral allograft transplantation, and meniscus allograft transplantation (MAT) provide alternatives to arthroplasty to help improve function and reduce pain.[15–31] In some settings, both cartilage restoration and arthroplasty may be viable surgical alternatives for these patients. Given that patients' status-post cartilage restoration can be revised to arthroplasty and arthroplasty cannot be revised back to native cartilage, cartilage restoration has been advocated as a "conservative" surgical approach that does not "burn any bridges."[15–31] If cartilage restoration fails, patients may progress to knee arthroplasty, including total knee arthroplasty (TKA) and

---

Disclosure Statement: The authors have nothing to disclose. The authors report that they have no conflicts of interest in the authorship and publication of this article.

Department of Orthopaedic Surgery, Rush University Medical Center, 1611 West Harrison, Suite 300, Chicago, IL 60612, USA

* Corresponding author.

E-mail address: rmfrank3@gmail.com

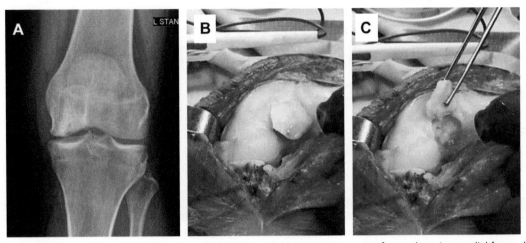

Fig. 1. A 39-year-old woman with continued left knee medial compartment pain after undergoing medial femoral condyle osteochondral allograft transplantation. (*A*) A 45° flexion weight-bearing posteroanterior radiograph demonstrating cystic changes of the left knee medial femoral condyle. (*B, C*) Osteochondral graft not healed at the time of unicompartmental knee arthroplasty, approximately 1.5 years following transplantation.

unicompartmental knee arthroplasty (UKA), as their definitive pain-relieving surgical solution. It remains unknown whether the outcome of knee arthroplasty after cartilage restoration is equivalent to the outcome had the knee arthroplasty been performed primarily.

To date, no data are available regarding clinical outcomes following conversion of a joint preservation procedure, such as cartilage/meniscal restoration, to TKA. Such information would be especially important with respect to preoperative counseling for patients related to the outcomes following arthroplasty procedures. Therefore, the purpose of this study was to compare the clinical outcomes of patients with a history of cartilage or meniscal restorative procedures with age-, sex-, and procedure-matched control patients undergoing primary TKA or UKA. The authors hypothesized that outcomes following primary TKA will be equivalent to those with TKA following cartilage and/or meniscus restoration.

METHODS

This study underwent approval by our university's institutional review board. A retrospective review of prospectively collected data on consecutive patients who underwent cartilage restoration by a single surgeon and subsequently progressed to arthroplasty was performed. Inclusion criteria included patients with a history of a prior open or arthroscopic cartilage and/or meniscal restoration procedure and subsequent ipsilateral UKA or TKA. The cartilage/meniscal restoration procedures included osteochondral autograft transfer, osteochondral allograft transplantation, and/or MAT of the same condyle and joint. All cartilage patients were matched with control patients based on sex, age ± 5 years, body mass index (BMI) ± 5, smoking status, and arthroplasty type. All patients in both the cartilage and the control groups were followed for a minimum of 2 years. Exclusion criteria in the cartilage group included patients whose cartilage/meniscal procedure was complicated by infection or chondrolysis as a complication of the index cartilage procedure and patients undergoing revision cartilage/meniscal restoration.

In the cartilage group, indications for cartilage/meniscal restoration versus primary knee arthroplasty included symptomatic, unipolar, full-thickness articular cartilage lesions and/or symptomatic meniscal deficiency not amenable to repair, in patients without diffuse arthritic changes in the affected compartment. Patients were also required to be ligamentously stable (or correctable) with neutral (or correctable) coronal plane alignment. In the cartilage group and the control groups, indications for arthroplasty were symptomatic medial or lateral tibiofemoral pain (UKA) or diffuse symptomatic bicompartmental or tricompartmental degenerative changes (TKA), unresponsive to prior treatment. In addition, indications for UKA included intact cruciate ligament status, lack of patellofemoral arthritis greater than grade III or IV on radiographs, lack of coronal plane deformity greater than 5°, and lack of knee flexion contracture greater than 5°. All patients in both groups underwent preoperative physical therapy.

Data collected for all patients included age, sex, laterality, comorbidities, preoperative and final follow-up Knee Society Score (KSS),[32–34] Quality of Life Short-Form-12 score, Hospital for Special Surgery scores, and range of motion (ROM). Prearthroplasty radiographs were graded according to the Kellgren and Lawrence scale.[35] In addition, the cartilage patients were assessed pre–cartilage procedure and post–cartilage procedure (prearthroplasty) with the following outcomes assessments: Tegner, Lysholm, International Knee Documentation Committee (IKDC), and Knee Injury and Osteoarthritis Outcome Score (KOOS) for pain. The control patients were not analyzed with the Tegner, Lysholm, IKDC, or KOOS scores because these outcomes instruments are not used in the preoperative or postoperative assessment of patients undergoing primary knee arthroplasty for osteoarthritis.

Statistical Analysis

All analyses were performed in Excel X (Microsoft Inc, Redmond, WA) and SPSS version 21 (IBM Inc, Armonk, NY). Categorical data were compared between study and control groups using chi-square and Fisher exact tests as appropriate. For continuous variables Komolgorov-Smirnov testing was performed. To compare between study and control groups Student t tests and Mann-Whitney U tests were performed as appropriate. Within study and control groups preoperative and postoperative data were compared using paired Student t tests and related-samples Wilcoxon signed rank tests as appropriate. Because a limited number of patients are available who have undergone both

cartilage restoration and knee arthroplasty on the same knee, all eligible patients were included and no a priori power analysis was conducted. A post hoc power analysis was performed; based on the means and standard deviations for the difference in preoperative and postoperative KSS the effect size was 1.67. With this study size the study's power was found to be 98%.

RESULTS

A total of 26 patients were included, with 13 patients (eight TKA and five UKA) in each group. The average clinical follow-up was 3.7 years (range, 2.0–7.2 years). There were no significant differences in age, sex, BMI, smoking status, worker's compensation status, preoperative physical therapy participation, preoperative ROM, postoperative ROM, or preoperative KSS scores between groups ($P>.05$ in all cases), suggesting adequate matching (Table 1). There were no intraoperative or postoperative complications, and there were no differences in tourniquet time between the cartilage and control groups (average of 82 vs 90 minutes, respectively; $P = .08$).

Before arthroplasty, the patients in the cartilage group underwent the following cartilage/meniscal restoration procedures: medial femoral condyle osteochondral allograft (n = 8), medial femoral condyle osteochondral allograft with corrective osteotomy (n = 1), MAT with anterior cruciate ligament reconstruction (n = 1), MAT with corrective osteotomy (n = 2), and patella osteochondral allograft with corrective osteotomy (n = 1). For the 10 patients with focal chondral lesions, the average defect size was

Table 1
Demographic data in the control group and the group status-post cartilage reconstruction

	Control Group	Cartilage Group	P Value
Age, y	44 ± 5	42 ± 6	.567
BMI	32 ± 7	31 ± 6	.576
Length of follow-up, y	3.3 ± 1.5	4 ± 1.7	.239
Time from cartilage restoration to arthroplasty, y	N/A	2.6 ± 1.8	N/A
Female, %	46	46	1.000
Smokers, %	15	15	1.000
Worker's compensation, %	23	38	.673
Arthroplasty type	5 UKA, 8 TKA	5 UKA, 8 TKA	N/A
Tourniquet time, min	90 ± 13	81 ± 10	.08

Data are displayed as means ± standard deviation.
Abbreviation: N/A, not applicable.

331 ± 204 mm² (range, 100–625 mm²). Before cartilage/meniscal restoration, patients had undergone an average 2 ± 2 prior surgeries (range, 1–7 surgeries) on the ipsilateral knee, including diagnostic arthroscopy, arthroscopic chondroplasty, arthroscopic partial meniscectomy, medial collateral ligament reconstruction, anterior cruciate ligament reconstruction, tibial plateau open reduction internal fixation, and medial patellofemoral ligament imbrication. Following cartilage/meniscal restoration, all patients underwent a standardized rehabilitation protocol at the direction of the senior author, including 6 to 8 weeks of protected weight-bearing, physical therapy, and return to full activities by 4 to 6 months following surgery. The duration of time between the cartilage/meniscal restoration procedure and the arthroplasty averaged 2.6 ± 1.8 years (range, 7.8 months to 7.7 years).

In the cartilage group, there were no significant differences in precartilage scores to postcartilage (prearthroplasty) scores for any of the outcomes assessments. Specifically, there were no postcartilage restoration improvements in the Tegner (2.4 ± 2.4–2.3 ± 0.8; P = .729), Lysholm (30.8 ± 17.1–38.2 ± 20.0; P = .474), IKDC (26.4 ± 10.3–33.0 ± 10.3; P = .847), or KOOS-pain (41.7 ± 19.4–59.0 ± 19.9; P = .672) scores.

Patients in the cartilage group had a significantly lower prearthroplasty (postcartilage) Kellgren and Lawrence grade (average, 2.6 ± 0.9) compared with matched control subjects (average, 3.7 ± 0.5; P = .004).

Patients in the cartilage group had significantly lower postoperative KSS scores (78 ± 13 vs 91 ± 5; P = .005) (Table 2) and experienced significantly less improvement in KSS scores (30 ± 10 vs 46 ± 10; P<.001). Two patients (15%) in the cartilage group required revision TKA at 1.9 years (for pain) and 4.7 years (for infection) following the index TKA. There were no reoperations in the control group.

DISCUSSION

Given the rise in the number of cartilage and meniscal restorative procedures being performed, it is important to understand the potential impact that these procedures may have on a subsequent arthroplasty. Our results suggest, that when compared with matched control subjects, patients undergoing arthroplasty after prior cartilage/meniscal restoration have significantly less pain relief, lower functional outcomes, and less improvement following UKA or TKA.

Patients undergoing cartilage and/or meniscal restoration procedures are difficult to treat. These patients are young, have high expectations, and have high activity levels. However, the surgical options for these patients are often salvage procedures, aimed at improving function for activities of daily living and relieving pain. Thus, the durability of joint preservation procedures may be limited. Arthroplasty is usually considered an option of last resort given the higher rates of complications and lower survivability of arthroplasty in young patients.[11,36–39] A recent study by Aggarwal and colleagues[11] compared 84 patients aged 50 years or younger with a sex- and BMI-matched cohort consisting of 84 patients aged 60 to 70 years (average, 62 years). Within the younger cohort revision TKA survivorship at 6 years was disappointingly low at 71%. Within this study, arthroplasty failure was more commonly attributed to aseptic loosening in the younger cohort and more commonly attributed to infection in the older cohort. The authors attributed these findings to younger patients being healthier and having a higher likelihood of subjecting their implants to higher levels of activities and loads. In the present study, we attempted to control for patient age to identify other potential risk factors for poor outcomes by matching both groups based on age, such that the average age for all patients (including the cartilage and the control groups) was 42 years, similar to the cohort in the Aggarwal study.[11]

Prior studies have suggested that, in general, prior knee surgery results in inferior outcomes following arthroplasty. Recently, Piedade and colleagues[40] reported on outcomes, complications, and failures in patients undergoing TKA after having undergone prior knee surgery (bone and soft tissue) compared with patients undergoing primary TKA alone (n = 1119). Prior procedures in the surgery group included bone procedures (n = 85), such as high tibial osteotomy, patellar realignment, and/or tibial plateau fracture surgery, and soft tissue procedures (n = 146), including arthroscopy and meniscectomy. At a minimum follow-up of 2 years, the authors reported worse postoperative flexion in the bone procedure group and a significantly increased complication rate in the soft tissue group, but an overall similar survivorship (and thus revision rate) in all three groups. In a separate study, the same group[41] reported in greater detail on the outcomes of the arthroscopy group (n = 60). Specifically, the authors reported a 30% local complication rate in the

Table 2
Outcome data in the control group and the group status-post cartilage reconstruction

	Control Group (n = 13)			Cartilage Group (n = 13)			Preoperative P Value	Postoperative P Value
	Preoperative	Postoperative	P Value	Preoperative	Postoperative	P Value		
Range of motion	110 ± 17	119 ± 10	.074	116 ± 17	117 ± 15	.872	.431	.703
Knee Society Score	45 ± 10	91 ± 5	<.001	48 ± 8	78 ± 13	<.001	.304	.005
Knee Society Score - Functional	47 ± 10	91 ± 6	<.001	50 ± 8	76 ± 20	<.001	.396	.016
Revised, %	N/A	0.00	N/A	N/A	15	N/A	N/A	N/A
With a complication, %	N/A	0.00	N/A	N/A	15	N/A	N/A	N/A

Data are displayed as means ± standard deviation.
Abbreviation: N/A, not applicable.

arthroscopy group, with 8.3% of those cases requiring revision TKA. Together, these reports indicate increased complications, but not necessarily worse overall clinical outcomes, in patients undergoing TKA after undergoing previous knee surgery. However, in these studies,[40,41] arthroplasty survivorship did not seem to be impacted by prior surgery. Longer follow-up is necessary to see if prior cartilage restoration impacts knee arthroplasty survivorship. To date, only a single study has analyzed outcomes in patients undergoing TKA after prior osteochondral allograft transplantation. In their cohort of 35 knees in 35 patients with an average age of 63 years, Morag and colleagues[42] reported improvements in KSS scores following arthroplasty at an average 92-month follow-up in 18 patients (KSS 45 preoperatively, KSS 82 postoperatively). Similar to the revision rate noted in our study, Morag and colleagues[42] described revision arthroplasty in six patients (17%) for aseptic loosening, with two revisions performed within 2 years following the index arthroplasty.

An important difference between the two groups of patients was that the control group had more severe disease preoperatively as measured by the Kellegren and Lawrence grade of their prearthroplasty radiographs. Other authors have shown a correlation between the severity of preoperative arthritis and final outcome following TKA.[43–45] Riis and colleagues[43] conducted a prospective study of 176 undergoing TKA and found that a low radiologic severity of osteoarthritis was associated with an inferior level of function ($P = .007$), but was not associated with pain. In a separate study, Dowsey and colleagues[45] evaluated 478 patients undergoing primary TKA and found that patients with a lower radiologic severity of arthritis at the time of arthroplasty were significantly more likely to report poor function and had significantly higher odds of postoperative moderate to severe pain ($P = .002$). Hence, it is important for surgeons to counsel patients preoperatively that the absence of full-thickness cartilage loss as seen on radiographs may be associated with a higher risk of dissatisfaction postoperatively.

Patients in the present study undergoing arthroplasty after prior cartilage/meniscal restoration still had significant improvements in KSS, despite lower preoperative Kellgren and Lawrence grades. In these patients, before arthroplasty, cartilage restoration did not improve functional outcomes, as evidenced by no clinical and statistical differences between preoperative and postoperative Tegner, Lysholm, IKDC, and

KOOS outcome scores. This is not typical of most cartilage restoration patients, who more commonly experience significant statistical and clinical improvements in these outcomes measures following cartilage and/or meniscal restoration.[12,46–49] Together, these findings suggest that knee arthroplasty is an effective procedure in patients who fail cartilage restoration, but that expectations must be tempered from the almost uniformly excellent outcomes that are achieved with primary knee arthroplasty.

This study has several limitations, including its small sample size, retrospective case-control design, and short-term follow-up. Our observations are not synonymous with cartilage restoration procedures being the sole cause of worse outcomes following revision to arthroplasty. Although increasing in overall incidence, cartilage restoration procedures are infrequently performed and even more infrequently revised to a knee arthroplasty, and thus large studies of this patient population are difficult to perform. A post hoc power analysis (based on KSS scores) demonstrated that the study is currently powered to 98% because the difference in outcomes between the groups is so large. The case-control design also introduces the potential for unmeasured residual bias between groups even though no significant differences were found between the groups preoperatively. A single patient in the cartilage group underwent revision arthroplasty because of infection, whereas no patients in the control group sustained an infection, and thus some of the differences in outcomes (especially reoperation rate) may be attributable to this factor. Of note, a second control group of patients undergoing cartilage restoration but without progression to arthroplasty was not evaluated as part of this study. The information that would be provided by such a control group was not thought to be relevant to the goal of this study, which was to determine how outcomes following knee arthroplasty are impacted by history of prior cartilage restoration, and instead would simply allow for the comparison of successful and failed cartilage restoration patients, which has been previously analyzed in a variety of cartilage/meniscal restoration studies.[15–31] Another limitation to this study is the relatively short-term follow-up, and certainly a study of longer-duration follow-up is necessary to see if these results are maintained over time.

Finally, and perhaps most important, patients undergoing arthroplasty for osteoarthritis (control subjects) may represent a different patient population compared with the patients undergoing arthroplasty for articular cartilage defects and thus the underlying diagnosis must be considered when extrapolating the results from this study to a specific patient. The purpose of this study was to determine whether the outcomes of arthroplasty performed for an indication of a failed cartilage procedure differ from the outcomes of arthroplasty performed for an indication of osteoarthritis. This information is useful prognostically and helps to guide knee arthroplasty expectations in patients with failed cartilage procedures. Underlying differences in preoperative indications, demographics, pathology, postoperative protocols, and numerous other factors likely play a role in outcomes determination, and thus the findings of this study cannot be used to determine whether cartilage restoration or arthroplasty provides superior outcomes for similar pathology. Notably, no patients in the control group underwent prior ipsilateral knee surgery, whereas patients in the cartilage group underwent an average of 2.2 prior ipsilateral knee surgeries, and although the number of prior knee surgeries may introduce bias, this is also typical of the cartilage patient population.

Explanations for why patients without osteoarthritis but who present with localized cartilage damage or following a functional meniscectomy have significant pain and functional limitations remain elusive. This coupled with the knowledge that patients with lesser degrees of arthritis have inferior outcomes following arthroplasty suggests that patients traditionally indicated for arthroplasty are inherently much different than those indicated for cartilage restoration. Identifying who will respond favorably among those who undergo cartilage restoration with minimal degrees of arthritis continues to be a significant knowledge gap among cartilage repair specialists.

SUMMARY

Although patients with a failed cartilage procedure do still derive benefit from knee arthroplasty, the magnitude of improvement and final scores are lower than matched control subjects. These patients also experienced little to no benefit from cartilage restoration, suggesting that unmeasured shared patient characteristics may play a role. This information can be used to counsel this difficult patient population on expected outcomes following arthroplasty procedures. Further research identifying characteristics of responders to treatment remains critical to refine clinical decision-making for this difficult patient group.

REFERENCES

1. Curl WW, Krome J, Gordon ES, et al. Cartilage injuries: a review of 31,516 knee arthroscopies. Arthroscopy 1997;13(4):456–60.
2. Hjelle K, Solheim E, Strand T, et al. Articular cartilage defects in 1,000 knee arthroscopies. Arthroscopy 2002;18(7):730–4.
3. Maletius W, Messner K. The effect of partial meniscectomy on the long-term prognosis of knees with localized, severe chondral damage. A twelve- to fifteen-year followup. Am J Sports Med 1996; 24(3):258–62.
4. Mankin HJ. The response of articular cartilage to mechanical injury. J Bone Joint Surg Am 1982; 64(3):460–6.
5. Messner K, Maletius W. The long-term prognosis for severe damage to weight-bearing cartilage in the knee: a 14-year clinical and radiographic follow-up in 28 young athletes. Acta Orthop Scand 1996;67(2):165–8.
6. Heir S, Nerhus TK, Rotterud JH, et al. Focal cartilage defects in the knee impair quality of life as much as severe osteoarthritis: a comparison of knee injury and osteoarthritis outcome score in 4 patient categories scheduled for knee surgery. Am J Sports Med 2010;38(2):231–7.
7. Gudas R, Kalesinskas RJ, Kimtys V, et al. A prospective randomized clinical study of mosaic osteochondral autologous transplantation versus microfracture for the treatment of osteochondral defects in the knee joint in young athletes. Arthroscopy 2005;21(9):1066–75.
8. Kon E, Gobbi A, Filardo G, et al. Arthroscopic second-generation autologous chondrocyte implantation compared with microfracture for chondral lesions of the knee: prospective nonrandomized study at 5 years. Am J Sports Med 2009;37(1):33–41.
9. Mithoefer K, Hambly K, Villa Della S, et al. Return to sports participation after articular cartilage repair in the knee: scientific evidence. Am J Sports Med 2009;37(Suppl 1):167S–76S.
10. Steadman JR, Miller BS, Karas SG, et al. The microfracture technique in the treatment of full-thickness chondral lesions of the knee in National Football League players. J Knee Surg 2003;16(2):83–6.
11. Aggarwal VK, Goyal N, Deirmengian G, et al. Revision total knee arthroplasty in the young patient: is there trouble on the horizon? J Bone Joint Surg Am 2014;96(7):536–42.
12. McCormick F, Harris JD, Abrams GD, et al. Survival and reoperation rates after meniscal allograft transplantation: analysis of failures for 172 consecutive transplants at a minimum 2-year follow-up. Am J Sports Med 2014;42(4):892–7.
13. McCormick F, Harris JD, Abrams GD, et al. Trends in the surgical treatment of articular cartilage

lesions in the United States: an analysis of a large private-payer database over a period of 8 years. Arthroscopy 2014;30(2):222–6.

14. Abrams GD, Frank RM, Gupta AK, et al. Trends in meniscus repair and meniscectomy in the United States, 2005-2011. Am J Sports Med 2013;41(10): 2333–9.

15. Gudas R, Stankevicius E, Monastyreckienė E, et al. Osteochondral autologous transplantation versus microfracture for the treatment of articular cartilage defects in the knee joint in athletes. Knee Surg Sports Traumatol Arthrosc 2006;14(9):834–42.

16. Kon E, Filardo G, Berruto M, et al. Articular cartilage treatment in high-level male soccer players: a prospective comparative study of arthroscopic second-generation autologous chondrocyte implantation versus microfracture. Am J Sports Med 2011;39(12):2549–57.

17. Basad E, Ishaque B, Bachmann G, et al. Matrix-induced autologous chondrocyte implantation versus microfracture in the treatment of cartilage defects of the knee: a 2-year randomised study. Knee Surg Sports Traumatol Arthrosc 2010;18(4):519–27.

18. Cerynik DL, Lewullis GE, Joves BC, et al. Outcomes of microfracture in professional basketball players. Knee Surg Sports Traumatol Arthrosc 2009;17(9): 1135–9.

19. Cole BJ, Farr J, Winalski CS, et al. Outcomes after a single-stage procedure for cell-based cartilage repair: a prospective clinical safety trial with 2-year follow-up. Am J Sports Med 2011;39(6):1170–9.

20. Ebert JR, Fallon M, Zheng MH, et al. A randomized trial comparing accelerated and traditional approaches to postoperative weightbearing rehabilitation after matrix-induced autologous chondrocyte implantation: findings at 5 years. Am J Sports Med 2012;40(7):1527–37.

21. Gooding CR, Bartlett W, Bentley G, et al. A prospective, randomised study comparing two techniques of autologous chondrocyte implantation for osteochondral defects in the knee: periosteum covered versus type I/III collagen covered. Knee 2006;13(3):203–10.

22. Horas U, Pelinkovic D, Herr G, et al. Autologous chondrocyte implantation and osteochondral cylinder transplantation in cartilage repair of the knee joint. A prospective, comparative trial. J Bone Joint Surg Am 2003;85A(2):185–92.

23. Knutsen G, Engebretsen L, Ludvigsen TC, et al. Autologous chondrocyte implantation compared with microfracture in the knee. A randomized trial. J Bone Joint Surg Am 2004;86A(3):455–64.

24. Kreuz PC, Steinwachs M, Erggelet C, et al. Importance of sports in cartilage regeneration after autologous chondrocyte implantation: a prospective study with a 3-year follow-up. Am J Sports Med 2007;35(8):1261–8.

25. Lim HC, Bae J-H, Song S-H, et al. Current treatments of isolated articular cartilage lesions of the knee achieve similar outcomes. Clin Orthop Relat Res 2012;470(8):2261–7.

26. Marder RA, Hopkins G, Timmerman LA. Arthroscopic microfracture of chondral defects of the knee: a comparison of two postoperative treatments. Arthroscopy 2005;21(2):152–8.

27. Niemeyer P, Köstler W, Salzmann GM, et al. Autologous chondrocyte implantation for treatment of focal cartilage defects in patients age 40 years and older: a matched-pair analysis with 2-year follow-up. Am J Sports Med 2010;38(12):2410–6.

28. Panagopoulos A, van Niekerk L, Triantafillopoulos I. Autologous chondrocyte implantation for knee cartilage injuries: moderate functional outcome and performance in patients with high-impact activities. Orthopedics 2012;35(1):e6–14.

29. Pestka JM, Bode G, Salzmann G, et al. Clinical outcome of autologous chondrocyte implantation for failed microfracture treatment of full-thickness cartilage defects of the knee joint. Am J Sports Med 2012;40(2):325–31.

30. Vanlauwe J, Saris DBF, Victor J, et al. Five-year outcome of characterized chondrocyte implantation versus microfracture for symptomatic cartilage defects of the knee: early treatment matters. Am J Sports Med 2011;39(12):2566–74.

31. Zaslav K, Cole B, Brewster R, et al. A prospective study of autologous chondrocyte implantation in patients with failed prior treatment for articular cartilage defect of the knee: results of the Study of the Treatment of Articular Repair (STAR) clinical trial. Am J Sports Med 2009; 37(1):42–55.

32. Ghanem E, Pawasarat I, Lindsay A, et al. Limitations of the Knee Society Score in evaluating outcomes following revision total knee arthroplasty. J Bone Joint Surg Am 2010;92(14):2445–51.

33. Insall JN, Dorr LD, Scott RD, et al. Rationale of the Knee Society clinical rating system. Clin Orthop Relat Res 1989;(248):13–4.

34. Liow RY, Walker K, Wajid MA, et al. The reliability of the American Knee Society Score. Acta Orthop Scand 2000;71(6):603–8.

35. Kellgren JH, Lawrence JS. Radiological assessment of osteo-arthrosis. Ann Rheum Dis 1957;16(4): 494–502.

36. Meehan JP, Danielsen B, Kim SH, et al. Younger age is associated with a higher risk of early peri-prosthetic joint infection and aseptic mechanical failure after total knee arthroplasty. J Bone Joint Surg Am 2014;96(7):529–35.

37. Stambough JB, Clohisy JC, Barrack RL, et al. Increased risk of failure following revision total knee replacement in patients aged 55 years and younger. Bone Joint J 2014;96B(12):1657–62.

38. W-Dahl A, Robertsson O, Lidgren L. Surgery for knee osteoarthritis in younger patients. Acta Orthop 2010;81(2):161–4.

39. Diduch DR, Insall JN, Scott WN, et al. Total knee replacement in young, active patients. Long-term follow-up and functional outcome. J Bone Joint Surg Am 1997;79(4):575–82.

40. Piedade SR, Pinaroli A, Servien E, et al. TKA outcomes after prior bone and soft tissue knee surgery. Knee Surg Sports Traumatol Arthrosc 2013;21(12):2737–43.

41. Piedade SR, Pinaroli A, Servien E, et al. Is previous knee arthroscopy related to worse results in primary total knee arthroplasty? Knee Surg Sports Traumatol Arthrosc 2009;17(4):328–33.

42. Morag G, Kulidjian A, Zalzal P, et al. Total knee replacement in previous recipients of fresh osteochondral allograft transplants. J Bone Joint Surg Am 2006;88(3):541–6.

43. Riis A, Rathleff MS, Jensen MB, et al. Low grading of the severity of knee osteoarthritis preoperatively is associated with a lower functional level after total knee replacement: a prospective cohort study with 12 months' follow-up. Bone Joint J 2014;96B(11):1498–502.

44. Dowsey MM, Dieppe P, Lohmander S, et al. The association between radiographic severity and pre-operative function in patients undergoing primary knee replacement for osteoarthritis. Knee 2012;19(6):860–5.

45. Dowsey MM, Nikpour M, Dieppe P, et al. Associations between pre-operative radiographic changes and outcomes after total knee joint replacement for osteoarthritis. Osteoarthr Cartil 2012;20(10):1095–102.

46. Chahal J, Gross AE, Gross C, et al. Outcomes of osteochondral allograft transplantation in the knee. Arthroscopy 2013;29(3):575–88.

47. Abrams GD, Hussey KE, Harris JD, et al. Clinical results of combined meniscus and femoral osteochondral allograft transplantation: minimum 2-year follow-up. Arthroscopy 2014;30(8):964–70.e1.

48. McCulloch PC, Kang RW, Sobhy MH, et al. Prospective evaluation of prolonged fresh osteochondral allograft transplantation of the femoral condyle: minimum 2-year follow-up. Am J Sports Med 2007;35(3):411–20.

49. Frank RM, Lee S, Levy D, et al. Osteochondral Allograft Transplantation of the Knee: Analysis of Failures at 5 Years. Am J Sports Med 2017;45(4):864–74.

Applications of Tissue Engineering in Joint Arthroplasty
Current Concepts Update

Hussein A. Zeineddine, MD[a], Todd J. Frush, MD[b],
Zeina M. Saleh, MD[c], Mouhanad M. El-Othmani, MD[d],
Khaled J. Saleh, MD, MSc, FRCS(C), MHCM, CPE[b],*

KEYWORDS

- Tissue engineering • Articular cartilage • Stem cells • Arthroplasty

---

KEY POINTS

- The technology of tissue engineering has witnessed substantial advancements and innovations in the recent years and carries significant potential for treating cartilaginous disorders.
- Although a variety of techniques in articular cartilage are available, preliminary data for almost all are encouraging.
- Several cell sources exist for tissue engineering; however, many parameters need further optimization, including the best-suited use of each cell source.
- Tissue engineering is already impacting clinical practice and will surely play an essential role in the daily practice in the foreseeable future.

INTRODUCTION

Cartilage is a highly specialized connective tissue maintained by chondrocytes. Articular cartilage is a highly organized tissue that is prone to undergo many alterations resulting from aging, trauma, or inflammatory processes, the end result of which is tissue deterioration, functional impairment, and pain.[1,2] Limited by the lack of vascularization and ability of migration of healthy chondrocytes to the damaged area, articular cartilage has a very limited ability to repair, making the management of the disease processes rather challenging.[3–5] Currently, total hip and total knee replacement are the preferred surgical interventions for end-stage arthritis.[6–8] More recently, tissue engineering and regenerative medicine have witnessed substantial advances, particularly with the introduction of new articular cartilage repair techniques.

Tissue engineering is a discipline aimed at restoring the functional role of various organs through the regeneration and formation of new tissues. It is being studied and applied in most organ systems, restoring the function of various tissues and organs, such as heart valves, blood vessels, the trachea, and bladder, among many others.[9–12] In general, tissue-engineering

---

Disclosures: No additional funding sources were used for this article.

Conflicts of Interest: No conflicts of interest are evident for authors of this article.

[a] Department of Surgery, University of Chicago Medical Center, 5841 South Maryland Avenue, Chicago, IL 60637, USA; [b] Department of Orthopaedics and Sports Medicine, Detroit Medical Center, University Health Center (UHC) 9B, 4201 Saint Antoine Street, Detroit, MI 48201-2153, USA; [c] Department of Surgery, American University of Beirut Medical Center, Bliss Street, Riad El-Solh, Beirut 11072020, Lebanon; [d] Department of Orthopaedics and Sports Medicine, Musculoskeletal Institute of Excellence, Detroit Medical Center, University Health Center (UHC) 9B, 4201 Saint Antoine Street, Detroit, MI 48201-2153, USA

* Corresponding author.

E-mail address: kjsaleh@gmail.com

http://dx.doi.org/10.1016/j.ocl.2017.03.002

application follows a general principle, albeit the presence of variances that occur within each step. The first step in tissue engineering is the proper choice of cells.[13–15] After being harvested, cells are cultured in vitro by placing them into a biomaterial scaffold that allows for cell differentiation or proliferation. The system is then placed in a bioreactor, which provides the necessary signals for proper development.[16] The tissue construct is finally implanted into the host (Fig. 1). The aforementioned protocol simplification serves as a model, and it should be reiterated that multiple variations of this general protocol exist, such as cell-free techniques, among others.[17,18] The purpose of this review is to present a current-concepts update on cell-based articular cartilage tissue engineering and briefly assess clinical trials using each cell source.

Chondrocyte-dependent Tissue Engineering

Various cell sources can be used in tissue engineering. A summary of the characteristics, main advantages, and disadvantages of each are presented in Tables 1 and 2. Chondrocytes, being the cells responsible for cartilage synthesis, have long been studied and used in articular tissue engineering.

Autologous chondrocyte implantation

Autologous chondrocyte implantation (ACI) was introduced in 1989[19] and was applied in the clinical setting in 1994 for treatment of deep cartilage defects of the knee.[20] Since its introduction, various clinical trials have been conducted to

assess the outcome and validity of the intervention. ACI is a 2-stage process:

1. First step, harvest and growth: arthroscopic excision of a biopsy from a healthy non-load- or low-load-bearing articular cartilage.
   a. Cartilage is then treated with enzymes in order to release chondrocytes.
   b. Followed by in vitro expansion to up to 48 million cells.
2. Second step, debridement and implantation: following the surgical debridement of the damaged cartilage, the chondrocytes are implanted into the injured area to healthy articular tissue and covered by a membrane, usually a periosteal flap or collagen sheet to void cell leakage.[2,21,22]

Various studies and trials reported positive short- and long-term follow-up outcomes with ACI technique.[23–27] However, with the current studies at hand,[28–30] the best use of ACI is still not well formulated. More work is needed to define the settings where ACI provides the best functional and/or financial outcome compared with the current standard treatments. The challenges that exist for ACI include prevention of cell leakage from the repair site and a high reoperation rate.

Chondrocyte-seeded scaffolds and matrix-induced autologous chondrocyte implantation

Similar to ACI, matrix-induced autologous chondrocyte implantation (MACI) is a 2-step procedure involving donor-site chondrocyte extraction

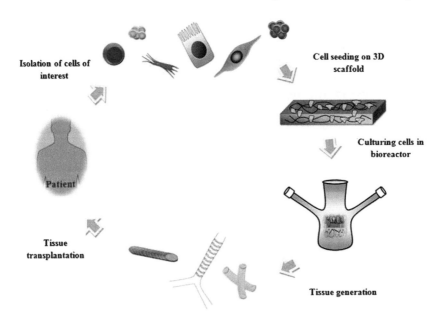

Fig. 1. General scheme for the process of tissue engineering.

Table 1
The characteristics of various cell sources that can be used in tissue engineering

Cell Source	Origin	Differentiation Capacity
Embryonic stem cells (ESC)	Blastocyst's inner cell mass	Cells of all 3 germ layers
iPS	Fibroblasts, hair follicle dermal papilla cells, umbilical vein endothelial cells, hepatocytes, melanocytes	Cells of all 3 germ layers
MSCs	Bone marrow, muscle, liver, umbilical cord blood, placenta and amnion, peripheral blood, pancreas, Wharton's jelly, brain, dental tissue, adipose tissue	Bone, cartilage, adipose tissue, muscle, neural, endothelial, insulin-producing cells
Very small embryonic-like stem cells	Bone marrow, cord blood, peripheral blood	Cells of all 3 germ layers
Direct conversion	Fibroblasts	Neurons, hepatocyte-like cells, multilineage blood progenitors, cardiomyocytes, macrophage-like cells
Terminally differentiated cells	Tissue of interest	—

followed by implantation. However, MACI uses an extra step in which the expanded chondrocytes are seeded into a 3-dimensional (3D) matrix made of porcine-derived mixed collagen (type I and III).[31] Chondrocyte-seeded scaffolds are numerous and include hyaluronan-based scaffolds,[32] bio-resorbable poly(lactic coglycolic acid) polymers,[33] and agarose-alginate hydrogel,[34] among many others.[35] In general, the use of scaffold aims at replicating the in vivo conditions in which the cells survive. This approach allows for the following:

1. Proper cellular growth and differentiation
2. Maintenance of the chondrogenic phenotype of the cells
3. Balanced and homogeneous distribution of chondrocytes and cartilage formation ensuring mechanical stability[36,37]

The tissue construct is thus more robust and capable of mimicking the crucial characteristics of the articular cartilage.[38,39] Although ACI requires cells to be injected, in scaffold-based

Table 2
The main advantages and disadvantages of various cell sources that can be used in tissue engineering

Cell Source	Advantages	Main Disadvantages and Challenges
Embryonic stem cells	Give rise to any cell type, unlimited proliferation	Scarce supply, ethical restrictions, immune compatibility
iPS	Give rise to any cell type, avoid host/donor incompatibility, production of patient-specific cell types, no ethical restrictions	Avoiding accumulation of environmental DNA damage, avoiding genetic modifications when using viral integration, target cell purification, efficiency of reprogramming, time consumption and costs, optimizing cell source for reprogramming, incomplete overlap with ESCs
MSCs	Give rise to a wide variety of cells, widely distributed and found, certain sources accessible with minimal invasive procedures, no ethical concerns, immune-compatible	Differentiation potential differs depending on origin, MSC lineage commitment dependent on various parameters to be resolved, phenotypic changes by prolonged passaging
Direct conversion	Direct generation of cells from fibroblasts with no need to revert to pluripotency	Limited cell types can be produced, time consuming, require further studies for optimization
Terminally differentiated cells	No need to induce differentiation, cells of interest already present	Scarce supply, limited proliferation capacity, cannot act as cell sources for tissues damaged by tumors

techniques, the cell-based scaffold is sutured or glued to the damaged cartilage. Although MACI has shown beneficial outcomes,[31] independent of the scaffold material used,[24,31,40,41] the procedure has not yet been proven superior to ACI or other standard interventions.[21,42–45] A recent systematic review asserted the need of more large-scale studies to dictate the optimal clinical application of MACI.[46]

ACI's most reported adverse effect is hypertrophy of the flap used in sealing the implanted cells.[2] Other adverse effects include postoperative pain as well as scar formation and limited mobility and fibroarthrosis secondary to the arthrotomy.[22,36,37] In addition, the need for a perifocal solid cartilage onto which the periosteal flap or collage sheet would be fixed narrows the applicability of ACI to focal cartilage lesions.[22] In contrast, scaffold-based MACI allows a better filling of the defect, is less technically challenging, has greater graft stability resulting in shorter recovery period, and can be used in diffuse defects when grafts can be fixed directly into subchondral bone.[2,22] Disadvantages of both techniques include cost, procedure complexity, and potential of chondrocyte dedifferentiation in culture into fibroblast-like cells.[47]

More recently, tissue engineering has been applying more prolonged forms of 3D seeding. In MACI, chondrocytes are seeded for 3 days, after which the tissue is implanted. This seeding technique might constitute an insufficient time for tissue organization, extracellular matrix (ECM) deposition, and achievement of biochemical integrity, rendering the tissue fragile and incompetent. To that end, new methods are implementing longer culturing periods, extending up to 6 weeks. The longer duration permits ample time for chondrocytes to proliferate, mature, deposit their own ECM, and achieve functional standards of mechanical robustness.[35,48] Aside from maintaining cells in their regular microenvironment of ECM, multiple confounding variables can impact the development and growth of cells, especially in terms of maintaining and inducing cellular differentiation. As chondrocytes expand in culture to achieve an adequate number of cells, the cells lose their chondrogenic phenotype with each passage. Minimizing dedifferentiation can be attained by decreasing the number of passages, optimizing expansion medium components (ie, growth factors), 3D culturing,[35,49–51] and exogenous mechanical stress.[52] The use of growth factors for chondrocyte expansion is an ongoing field of research. FGF-2 has been shown to maintain chondrogenic phenotype, induce proliferation, and promote neocartilage with higher matrix content.[53–55] Many other factors have been reported to play a pivotal role in chondrocyte proliferation and differentiation, including EGF, TGF-B1, and BMPs, among others.[56–60] Scaffolds used in cartilage tissue engineering are numerous and beyond the scope of this review. However, such scaffolds are generally divided into microporous (hydrogels) and macroporous scaffolds, each with its own advantages and disadvantages.[35] Biomemetic stimuli are also known to play integral roles in chondrocyte differentiation and development. A main exogenous stimulus in 3D culture is mechanical stimulation. Cartilage endures mechanical stress and continuous load bearing, and thus, the designed neotissue must be able to mirror this capacity and withhold regular joint loads. Chondrocytes are known to proliferate and produce more ECM in response to mechanical loads, such as hydrostatic pressure and dynamic compression, among others.[52,60–65] However, applying mechanical stimuli in a consistent manner and in large scale remains a technical challenge.[35] Other relevant exogenous stimuli include hypoxia, which increases ECM deposition and improves the biochemical properties of collagen,[66,67] pH,[68] direct perfusion,[69] the use of chemicals and enzymes,[35,70] and coculturing with mesenchymal stem cells (MSCs).[71,72]

Scaffold-free technologies rely on culturing chondrocytes at high densities. Over a couple of weeks, cells secrete ECM while adhering together,[73,74] which results in forming the final robust neotissue. Stimulation of these constructs with exogenous stimuli has been shown to result in tissue with similar properties and qualities of normal in vivo cartilage.[2,67,70,75] Clinical trials are being conducted on both Chondrosphere (Teltow, Germany) and RevaFle (St. Louis, MO, USA), the 2 main scaffold-free constructs.

Stem Cell-based Tissue Engineering

Chondrocyte-dependent cartilage regeneration remains costly and invasive and carries the risk of dedifferentiation into a fibroblast-like stage. Thus, stem cells have been explored as an alternative source of cells.

Mesenchymal stem cells

MSCs hold a true promise for tissue engineering. MSCs are capable of differentiating into bone, cartilage, adipose tissue, muscle, neural, endothelial, and insulin-producing cells.[76–80] MSCs retain their multilineage differentiation potential in culture with an extensive proliferative ability in an uncommitted state.[81] "Mesenchymal stem cells" is a terminology used to refer to stromal cells with specific properties. The International Society for Cellular Therapy proposed a standard set of rules to define the identity of these cells[82]:

1. MSCs should be plastic adherent, forming fibroblast-like colonies
2. MSCs should be able to differentiate into various specialized cell lineages
3. Ability to express defined cell surface marker profiles

Although there is a no definite set of markers, the agreed upon markers of MSCs include specific immunophenotypic marker combinations (CD73, CD90, and CD105) and lack both hematopoietic markers (CD11b, CD19, CD34, and CD45) and class II major histocompatibility complex (MHC) molecules (HLA-DR).[82] MSCs have various sources such as bone marrow (BM-MSCs), muscle, liver, synovium, umbilical cord blood (UC-MSCs), placenta and amnion, peripheral blood, pancreas, dental tissue, adipose tissue (ASCs), and urine.[79,83–88] The wide variety and large number of sources, capability of differentiating into various types of specific-cell lineages, minimal ethical concerns, and immune-compatibility make MSCs a robust viable option in tissue engineering and regenerative medicine.

Bone marrow mesenchymal stem cells

BM-MSCs are the most studied MSCs for cartilage tissue engineering. BM-MSCs from a diseased individual have been shown to produce cartilage similar to that of healthy MSCs donors and maintain the chondrogenic phenotype in the presence of TGf-b.[37,89] As well, BM-MSCs have been shown to maintain an anti-inflammatory state in diseased organs.[90] In general, these cells have been implemented in the clinical setting in 2 ways:

1. Intra-articular injection of the cells
2. Using an MACI-like approach

The beneficial outcomes of intra-articular injection have been reported in preclinical studies, case series, as well as randomized studies.[91–97] The MACI-like technique has also shown promising results, albeit less evidence and support in the literature. Culturing BM-MSCs on scaffolds before implantation has shown good functional outcomes in several studies.[98–102] However, some studies also noted no benefit of BM-MSC's administration per se when used as an add-on to the current standard procedure of microfracture. Nevertheless, the beneficial effect stems from the minimal invasive technique used in the BM-MSC group.[103]

In summary, the use of BM-MSCs has been showing substantial promise. Direct injection of BM-MSCs into diseased cartilage has shown beneficial outcomes comparable to ACI, with the added benefit of being less costly and avoiding the risk of an additional surgery and donor site morbidity. However, many parameters still need to be optimized, including dosing regimens, and results of current and further trials must be analyzed to ensure safety of MSCs, effectiveness over the long-term and comparative efficacy to other available treatments.

Umbilical cord derived mesenchymal stem cells

Umbilical cord blood has been shown to contain stem cells with mesenchymal properties[104,105] capable of differentiating into various cell types including chondrocytes.[106,107] Collection of umbilical cord derived MSCs (UC-MSCs) is noninvasive and relatively easy, with not much of an ethical debate generated.[108] To date, no human clinical trial was conducted to assess the efficacy of cartilage generated using UC-MSCs. However, results of a limited number of preclinical studies seem encouraging. In one study, using UC-MSCs with a hyaluronic acid hydrogel composite in minipigs resulted in a superior and more complete hyaline cartilage regeneration than the control group.[109] Another study using rat models also showed significant improvement in the knee receiving UC-MSCs compared with the contralateral one.[110] Although UC-MSCs are showing positive results in preclinical trials, it is still too early to draw a conclusion, especially with the lack of human clinical trials.

Adipose tissue–derived mesenchymal stem cells

ASCs have been regarded as a desirable cell choice for various reasons:

1. Readily accessible
2. Availability in large quantities

3. Capability of differentiation similar to BM-MSCs
4. Lack of immunogenicity
5. Anti-inflammatory properties
6. Minimal ethical considerations[111–113]

In a study of 18 patients, intra-articular injection of ASCs resulted in improved function and pain of the knee joint with documented regeneration of hyaline-like articular cartilage.[114] The beneficial effects of ASCs on cartilage regeneration were also evident in 3 other trials, with a total of 133 patients.[115–117] One of the studies found improved results of scaffold-based ASCs compared with ASCs injection alone.[115] Other early studies have shown improvement in validated outcomes scores and pain scores but have not shown evidence of cartilage regeneration, one of the primary goals of stem cell technology. The feasibility and positive outcomes of ASCs injection were also documented in a study of an elderly population with cartilage healing, functional improvement, and pain reduction.[118] Similar to BM-MSCs, although initial results are encouraging, more research and trials should be invested in this promising technology.

Peripheral blood–derived mesenchymal stem cells

Peripheral blood has been found to be a source of MSCs capable of differentiating into chondrocytes.[119] Even though limited in number, the effect of PB-MSCs on cartilage repair has been largely positive in all clinical trials conducted so far. The earliest study was conducted in 2011 on 5 patients, showing the proof of concept of using PB-MSCs for cartilage repair.[120] Following that, 4 more clinical trials were conducted,[121–124] demonstrating beneficial effects with clinical improvement and histologic evidence of substantial deposition of chondrogenic ECM.

Synovial-derived mesenchymal stem cells

In vitro and preclinical studies had shown the differentiation capacity as well as the beneficial effect of synovial-derived MSCs on cartilage repair.[125–128] Human trials however had been limited. In one study, clinical outcome was improved, and documented healing was observed on MRI and second-look arthroscopy.[129] Interestingly, the second trial showed a significant improvement using synovial-derived MSCs compared with MACI.[130] However, this trial had a relatively small sample size of only 14 participants.

Other mesenchymal stem cells

Other tissue sources have been reported to harbor cells with chondrogenic differentiation potential.[131] These other tissue sources include dermal stem cells,[132,133] muscle-derived MSCs,[134] placenta-derived MSCs,[135] ear elastic cartilage,[136] and periosteum.[137,138]

Induced Pluripotent Stem Cells

Induced pluripotent stem cells (iPS) are autologous, somatic cells that undergo nuclear reprogramming into a primordial, embryonic stem cell–like state.[139] iPS cells have the hallmarks of ES cell, including the following:

1. Morphology
2. Unlimited self-renewal
3. Expression of key pluripotency genes
4. Normal karyotype

In addition, human iPS cells have been proven to undergo functional differentiation into specialized cell lineages of all 3 embryonic germ layers. Reprogramming aims to induce differentiated cells to reverting to pluripotency. Once pluripotency is achieved, differentiation into almost any cell type can be achieved.[140] The initial description of generating iPS was from Yamanaka in which introducing only 4 transcription factors (Oct3/4, c-Myc, Sox2, and Klf4) reprogrammed mouse adult fibroblasts into a pluripotent state.[141–143] Following that, a variety of cells were used to induce pluripotency using different methods, including hair follicle dermal papillae,[144] umbilical vein endothelial cells,[145] hepatocytes,[146] melanocytes,[147] adipose tissue,[148] peripheral blood cell,[149,150] and many others.[151] iPS were shown to differentiate into cartilage in vitro and actually had proven beneficial effect in preclinical studies.[152–154] Although promising, evidence supporting iPS is still in an early stage compared with other cell sources. Many issues need to be resolved, including the differentiation capacity and chondrogenic phenotype in the long run, the potential for teratogenesis, resolving any carry-over undesired "epigenetic memory"[155] and further in vivo testing.

DIRECT LINEAGE CONVERSION

More recently, scientists were able to induce cell-to-cell differentiation directly, bypassing the need to induce a pluripotent state. Direct conversion currently uses fibroblasts as the cell source and has been shown to be able to produce macrophages,[156] neuronal cells,[157–160] hepatocytes,[161] multilineage blood cells,[162] and cardiomyocytes.[163,164] Fibroblasts have also been directly converted into chondrocytes with documented chondrogenic ECM deposition.[165,166] In one pioneering study implementing direct conversion using cell sources other than fibroblasts, placental-derived cells were used for direct conversion into chondrocytes.[167] The advent of transdifferentiation is certainly a critical step in the advances of tissue engineering; however, further research and investigation are required before being able to take it from the bench side to rigorous in vivo studies.

SUMMARY

This review focused on tissue engineering techniques for cartilage repair that uses cell sources. However, other cell-free techniques are already being applied for cartilage repair. The technology of tissue engineering has witnessed substantial advancements and innovations in recent years and carries significant potential for treating cartilaginous disorders. Although much work is still required to truly develop and mimic the native human cartilage with its various aspects, this goal is much closer to reality with each day.

REFERENCES

1. Vinatier C, Guicheux J. Cartilage tissue engineering: from biomaterials and stem cells to osteoarthritis treatments. Ann Phys Rehabil Med 2016; 59(3):139–44.
2. Makris EA, Gomoll AH, Malizos KN, et al. Repair and tissue engineering techniques for articular cartilage. Nat Rev Rheumatol 2015;11(1):21–34.
3. Jones DG, Peterson L. Autologous chondrocyte implantation. J Bone Joint Surg Am 2006;88(11): 2502–20.
4. Cole BJ, Pascual-Garrido C, Grumet RC. Surgical management of articular cartilage defects in the knee. J Bone Joint Surg Am 2009;91(7):1778–90.
5. Mankin HJ. The response of articular cartilage to mechanical injury. J Bone Joint Surg Am 1982; 64(3):460–6.
6. Mahomed NN, Barrett JA, Katz JN, et al. Rates and outcomes of primary and revision total hip replacement in the United States Medicare population. J Bone Joint Surg Am 2003;85-A(1):27–32.
7. Hawker G, Wright J, Coyte P, et al. Health-related quality of life after knee replacement. J Bone Joint Surg Am 1998;80(2):163–73.
8. Mandl LA. Determining who should be referred for total hip and knee replacements. Nat Rev Rheumatol 2013;9(6):351–7.

9. Kusuma S, Gerecht S. Engineering blood vessels using stem cells: innovative approaches to treat vascular disorders. Expert Rev Cardiovasc Ther 2010;8(10):1433–45.

10. Siemionow M, Bozkurt M, Zor F. Regeneration and repair of peripheral nerves with different biomaterials: review. Microsurgery 2010;30(7):574–88.

11. Sun H, Liu W, Zhou G, et al. Tissue engineering of cartilage, tendon and bone. Front Med 2011; 5(1):61–9.

12. Shin YS, Choi JW, Park JK, et al. Tissue-engineered tracheal reconstruction using mesenchymal stem cells seeded on a porcine cartilage powder scaffold. Ann Biomed Eng 2015;43(4): 1003–13.

13. Stocum DL, Zupanc GK. Stretching the limits: stem cells in regeneration science. Dev Dyn 2008;237(12):3648–71.

14. Togel F, Westenfelder C. Adult bone marrow-derived stem cells for organ regeneration and repair. Dev Dyn 2007;236(12):3321–31.

15. Sundelacruz S, Kaplan DL. Stem cell- and scaffold-based tissue engineering approaches to osteochondral regenerative medicine. Semin Cell Dev Biol 2009;20(6):646–55.

16. Howard D, Buttery LD, Shakesheff KM, et al. Tissue engineering: strategies, stem cells and scaffolds. J Anat 2008;213(1):66–72.

17. Kusano T, Jakob RP, Gautier E, et al. Treatment of isolated chondral and osteochondral defects in the knee by autologous matrix-induced chondrogenesis (AMIC). Knee Surg Sports Traumatol Arthrosc 2012;20(10):2109–15.

18. Benthien JP, Behrens P. The treatment of chondral and osteochondral defects of the knee with autologous matrix-induced chondrogenesis (AMIC): method description and recent developments. Knee Surg Sports Traumatol Arthrosc 2011;19(8):1316–9.

19. Grande DA, Pitman MI, Peterson L, et al. The repair of experimentally produced defects in rabbit articular cartilage by autologous chondrocyte transplantation. J Orthop Res 1989;7(2): 208–18.

20. Brittberg M, Lindahl A, Nilsson A, et al. Treatment of deep cartilage defects in the knee with autologous chondrocyte transplantation. N Engl J Med 1994;331(14):889–95.

21. Bartlett W, Skinner JA, Gooding CR, et al. Autologous chondrocyte implantation versus matrix-induced autologous chondrocyte implantation for osteochondral defects of the knee: a prospective, randomised study. J Bone Joint Surg Br 2005; 87(5):640–5.

22. Ringe J, Burmester GR, Sittinger M. Regenerative medicine in rheumatic disease-progress in tissue engineering. Nat Rev Rheumatol 2012;8(8):493–8.

23. Saris DB, Vanlauwe J, Victor J, et al. Treatment of symptomatic cartilage defects of the knee: characterized chondrocyte implantation results in better clinical outcome at 36 months in a randomized trial compared to microfracture. Am J Sports Med 2009;37(Suppl 1):10S–9S.

24. Saris DB, Vanlauwe J, Victor J, et al. Characterized chondrocyte implantation results in better structural repair when treating symptomatic cartilage defects of the knee in a randomized controlled trial versus microfracture. Am J Sports Med 2008;36(2):235–46.

25. Peterson L, Vasiliadis HS, Brittberg M, et al. Autologous chondrocyte implantation: a long-term follow-up. Am J Sports Med 2010;38(6):1117–24.

26. Minas T, Von Keudell A, Bryant T, et al. The John Insall Award: a minimum 10-year outcome study of autologous chondrocyte implantation. Clin Orthop Relat Res 2014;472(1):41–51.

27. Behery OA, Harris JD, Karnes JM, et al. Factors influencing the outcome of autologous chondrocyte implantation: a systematic review. J Knee Surg 2013;26(3):203–11.

28. Bentley G, Biant LC, Vijayan S, et al. Minimum ten-year results of a prospective randomised study of autologous chondrocyte implantation versus mosaicplasty for symptomatic articular cartilage lesions of the knee. J Bone Joint Surg Br 2012; 94(4):504–9.

29. Van Assche D, Staes F, Van Caspel D, et al. Autologous chondrocyte implantation versus microfracture for knee cartilage injury: a prospective randomized trial, with 2-year follow-up. Knee Surg Sports Traumatol Arthrosc 2010;18(4): 486–95.

30. Knutsen G, Drogset JO, Engebretsen L, et al. A randomized trial comparing autologous chondrocyte implantation with microfracture. Findings at five years. J Bone Joint Surg Am 2007;89(10): 2105–12.

31. Behrens P, Bitter T, Kurz B, et al. Matrix-associated autologous chondrocyte transplantation/implantation (MACT/MACI)–5-year follow-up. Knee 2006; 13(3):194–202.

32. Nehrer S, Domayer S, Dorotka R, et al. Three-year clinical outcome after chondrocyte transplantation using a hyaluronan matrix for cartilage repair. Eur J Radiol 2006;57(1):3–8.

33. Sha'ban M, Kim SH, Idrus RB, et al. Fibrin and poly(lactic-co-glycolic acid) hybrid scaffold promotes early chondrogenesis of articular chondrocytes: an in vitro study. J Orthop Surg Res 2008;3:17.

34. Selmi TA, Verdonk P, Chambat P, et al. Autologous chondrocyte implantation in a novel alginate-agarose hydrogel: outcome at two years. J Bone Joint Surg Br 2008;90(5):597–604.

35. Huang BJ, Hu JC, Athanasiou KA. Cell-based tissue engineering strategies used in the clinical repair of articular cartilage. Biomaterials 2016; 98:1–22.

36. Sittinger M, Burmester GR. Can engineered cartilage transplants be used for treating rheumatic diseases? Nat Clin Pract Rheumatol 2006;2(4): 172–3.

37. Ringe J, Sittinger M. Tissue engineering in the rheumatic diseases. Arthritis Res Ther 2009; 11(1):211.

38. Moutos FT, Guilak F. Composite scaffolds for cartilage tissue engineering. Biorheology 2008; 45(3–4):501–12.

39. Zhang L, Hu J, Athanasiou KA. The role of tissue engineering in articular cartilage repair and regeneration. Crit Rev Biomed Eng 2009;37(1–2):1–57.

40. Kon E, Di Martino A, Filardo G, et al. Second-generation autologous chondrocyte transplantation: MRI findings and clinical correlations at a minimum 5-year follow-up. Eur J Radiol 2011;79(3): 382–8.

41. Ossendorf C, Kaps C, Kreuz PC, et al. Treatment of posttraumatic and focal osteoarthritic cartilage defects of the knee with autologous polymer-based three-dimensional chondrocyte grafts: 2-year clinical results. Arthritis Res Ther 2007;9(2):R41.

42. Marlovits S, Aldrian S, Wondrasch B, et al. Clinical and radiological outcomes 5 years after matrix-induced autologous chondrocyte implantation in patients with symptomatic, traumatic chondral defects. Am J Sports Med 2012;40(10):2273–80.

43. Zheng MH, Willers C, Kirilak L, et al. Matrix-induced autologous chondrocyte implantation (MACI): biological and histological assessment. Tissue Eng 2007;13(4):737–46.

44. Zeifang F, Oberle D, Nierhoff C, et al. Autologous chondrocyte implantation using the original periosteum-cover technique versus matrix-associated autologous chondrocyte implantation: a randomized clinical trial. Am J Sports Med 2010; 38(5):924–33.

45. Ebert JR, Robertson WB, Woodhouse J, et al. Clinical and magnetic resonance imaging-based outcomes to 5 years after matrix-induced autologous chondrocyte implantation to address articular cartilage defects in the knee. Am J Sports Med 2011;39(4):753–63.

46. Kon E, Filardo G, Di Matteo B, et al. Matrix assisted autologous chondrocyte transplantation for cartilage treatment: a systematic review. Bone JointRes 2013;2(2):18–25.

47. Dehne T, Karlsson C, Ringe J, et al. Chondrogenic differentiation potential of osteoarthritic chondrocytes and their possible use in matrix-associated autologous chondrocyte transplantation. Arthritis Res Ther 2009;11(5):R133.

48. Smeriglio P, Lai JH, Yang F, et al. 3D hydrogel scaffolds for articular chondrocyte culture and cartilage generation. J Vis Exp 2015;104:1–6.

49. Caron MM, Emans PJ, Coolsen MM, et al. Redifferentiation of dedifferentiated human articular chondrocytes: comparison of 2D and 3D cultures. Osteoarthritis Cartilage 2012;20(10):1170–8.

50. Mandl EW, van der Veen SW, Verhaar JA, et al. Serum-free medium supplemented with high-concentration FGF2 for cell expansion culture of human ear chondrocytes promotes redifferentiation capacity. Tissue Eng 2002;8(4):573–80.

51. Mandl EW, van der Veen SW, Verhaar JA, et al. Multiplication of human chondrocytes with low seeding densities accelerates cell yield without losing redifferentiation capacity. Tissue Eng 2004; 10(1–2):109–18.

52. Jeon JE, Schrobback K, Hutmacher DW, et al. Dynamic compression improves biosynthesis of human zonal chondrocytes from osteoarthritis patients. Osteoarthritis Cartilage 2012;20(8): 906–15.

53. Mandl EW, Jahr H, Koevoet JL, et al. Fibroblast growth factor-2 in serum-free medium is a potent mitogen and reduces dedifferentiation of human ear chondrocytes in monolayer culture. Matrix Biol 2004;23(4):231–41.

54. Martin I, Suetterlin R, Baschong W, et al. Enhanced cartilage tissue engineering by sequential exposure of chondrocytes to FGF-2 during 2D expansion and BMP-2 during 3D cultivation. J Cell Biochem 2001;83(1):121–8.

55. Yang KG, Saris DB, Geuze RE, et al. Impact of expansion and redifferentiation conditions on chondrogenic capacity of cultured chondrocytes. Tissue Eng 2006;12(9):2435–47.

56. Vivien D, Galera P, Lebrun E, et al. Differential effects of transforming growth factor-beta and epidermal growth factor on the cell cycle of cultured rabbit articular chondrocytes. J Cell Physiol 1990;143(3):534–45.

57. Shepard JB, Jeong JW, Maihle NJ, et al. Transient anabolic effects accompany epidermal growth factor receptor signal activation in articular cartilage in vivo. Arthritis Res Ther 2013;15(3):R60.

58. van der Kraan P, Vitters E, van den Berg W. Differential effect of transforming growth factor beta on freshly isolated and cultured articular chondrocytes. J Rheumatol 1992;19(1):140–5.

59. Hwang NS, Kim MS, Sampattavanich S, et al. Effects of three-dimensional culture and growth factors on the chondrogenic differentiation of murine embryonic stem cells. Stem Cells 2006;24(2):284–91.

60. Elder BD, Athanasiou KA. Systematic assessment of growth factor treatment on biochemical and

biomechanical properties of engineered articular cartilage constructs. Osteoarthritis Cartilage 2009;17(1):114–23.

61. Appelman TP, Mizrahi J, Elisseeff JH, et al. The influence of biological motifs and dynamic mechanical stimulation in hydrogel scaffold systems on the phenotype of chondrocytes. Biomaterials 2011;32(6):1508–16.

62. Mizuno S, Tateishi T, Ushida T, et al. Hydrostatic fluid pressure enhances matrix synthesis and accumulation by bovine chondrocytes in three-dimensional culture. J Cell Physiol 2002;193(3): 319–27.

63. Smith RL, Rusk SF, Ellison BE, et al. In vitro stimulation of articular chondrocyte mRNA and extracellular matrix synthesis by hydrostatic pressure. J Orthop Res 1996;14(1):53–60.

64. Hasanova GI, Noriega SE, Mamedov TG, et al. The effect of ultrasound stimulation on the gene and protein expression of chondrocytes seeded in chitosan scaffolds. J Tissue Eng Regen Med 2011;5(10):815–22.

65. Xu X, Urban JP, Tirlapur UK, et al. Osmolarity effects on bovine articular chondrocytes during three-dimensional culture in alginate beads. Osteoarthritis Cartilage 2010;18(3):433–9.

66. Meretoja VV, Dahlin RL, Wright S, et al. The effect of hypoxia on the chondrogenic differentiation of co-cultured articular chondrocytes and mesenchymal stem cells in scaffolds. Biomaterials 2013; 34(17):4266–73.

67. Makris EA, Hu JC, Athanasiou KA. Hypoxia-induced collagen crosslinking as a mechanism for enhancing mechanical properties of engineered articular cartilage. Osteoarthritis Cartilage 2013;21(4):634–41.

68. Das RH, van Osch GJ, Kreukniet M, et al. Effects of individual control of pH and hypoxia in chondrocyte culture. J Orthop Res 2010;28(4):537–45.

69. Gharravi AM, Orazizadeh M, Hashemitabar M. Direct expansion of chondrocytes in a dynamic three-dimensional culture system: overcoming dedifferentiation effects in monolayer culture. Artif Organs 2014;38(12):1053–8.

70. Makris EA, MacBarb RF, Paschos NK, et al. Combined use of chondroitinase-ABC, TGF-beta1, and collagen crosslinking agent lysyl oxidase to engineer functional neotissues for fibrocartilage repair. Biomaterials 2014;35(25):6787–96.

71. Meretoja VV, Dahlin RL, Kasper FK, et al. Enhanced chondrogenesis in co-cultures with articular chondrocytes and mesenchymal stem cells. Biomaterials 2012;33(27):6362–9.

72. Meretoja VV, Dahlin RL, Wright S, et al. Articular chondrocyte redifferentiation in 3D co-cultures with mesenchymal stem cells. Tissue Eng C Methods 2014;20(6):514–23.

73. Athanasiou KA, Eswaramoorthy R, Hadidi P, et al. Self-organization and the self-assembling process in tissue engineering. Annu Rev Biomed Eng 2013; 15:115–36.

74. DuRaine GD, Brown WE, Hu JC, et al. Emergence of scaffold-free approaches for tissue engineering musculoskeletal cartilages. Ann Biomed Eng 2015;43(3):543–54.

75. Gunja NJ, Uthamanthil RK, Athanasiou KA. Effects of TGF-beta1 and hydrostatic pressure on meniscus cell-seeded scaffolds. Biomaterials 2009;30(4):565–73.

76. Griffin M, Iqbal SA, Bayat A. Exploring the application of mesenchymal stem cells in bone repair and regeneration. J Bone Joint Surg Br 2011; 93(4):427–34.

77. Pittenger MF, Mackay AM, Beck SC, et al. Multilineage potential of adult human mesenchymal stem cells. Science 1999;284(5411):143–7.

78. Kim EY, Lee KB, Yu J, et al. Neuronal cell differentiation of mesenchymal stem cells originating from canine amniotic fluid. Hum Cell 2014;27(2):51–8.

79. Manochantr S, Tantrawatpan C, Kheolamai P, et al. Isolation, characterization and neural differentiation potential of amnion derived mesenchymal stem cells. J Med Assoc Thai 2010; 93(Suppl 7):S183–91.

80. Oswald J, Boxberger S, Jorgensen B, et al. Mesenchymal stem cells can be differentiated into endothelial cells in vitro. Stem Cells 2004; 22(3):377–84.

81. Augello A, Kurth TB, De Bari C. Mesenchymal stem cells: a perspective from in vitro cultures to in vivo migration and niches. Eur Cell Mater 2010;20:121–33.

82. Horwitz EM, Le Blanc K, Dominici M, et al. Clarification of the nomenclature for MSC: the International Society for Cellular Therapy position statement. Cytotherapy 2005;7(5):393–5.

83. Seeberger KL, Eshpeter A, Korbutt GS. Isolation and culture of human multipotent stromal cells from the pancreas. Methods Mol Biol 2011;698: 123–40.

84. Zhang D, Wei G, Li P, et al. Urine-derived stem cells: a novel and versatile progenitor source for cell-based therapy and regenerative medicine. Genes Dis 2014;1(1):8–17.

85. Estrela C, Alencar AH, Kitten GT, et al. Mesenchymal stem cells in the dental tissues: perspectives for tissue regeneration. Braz Dent J 2011; 22(2):91–8.

86. Mihu CM, Mihu D, Costin N, et al. Isolation and characterization of stem cells from the placenta and the umbilical cord. Rom J Morphol Embryol 2008;49(4):441–6.

87. Tsagias N, Koliakos I, Karagiannis V, et al. Isolation of mesenchymal stem cells using the total

length of umbilical cord for transplantation purposes. Transfus Med 2011;21(4):253–61.

88. Hass R, Kasper C, Bohm S, et al. Different populations and sources of human mesenchymal stem cells (MSC): a comparison of adult and neonatal tissue-derived MSC. Cell Commun Signal 2011;9:12.

89. Kafienah W, Mistry S, Dickinson SC, et al. Three-dimensional cartilage tissue engineering using adult stem cells from osteoarthritis patients. Arthritis Rheum 2007;56(1):177–87.

90. Zhang Y, Pizzute T, Pei M. Anti-inflammatory strategies in cartilage repair. Tissue Eng B Rev 2014; 20(6):655–68.

91. Vangsness CT Jr, Farr J 2nd, Boyd J, et al. Adult human mesenchymal stem cells delivered via intra-articular injection to the knee following partial medial meniscectomy: a randomized, double-blind, controlled study. J Bone Joint Surg Am 2014;96(2):90–8.

92. Emadedin M, Aghdami N, Taghiyar L, et al. Intra-articular injection of autologous mesenchymal stem cells in six patients with knee osteoarthritis. Arch Iran Med 2012;15(7):422–8.

93. Centeno CJ, Busse D, Kisiday J, et al. Increased knee cartilage volume in degenerative joint disease using percutaneously implanted, autologous mesenchymal stem cells. Pain Physician 2008; 11(3):343–53.

94. Nejadnik H, Hui JH, Feng Choong EP, et al. Autologous bone marrow-derived mesenchymal stem cells versus autologous chondrocyte implantation: an observational cohort study. Am J Sports Med 2010;38(6):1110–6.

95. Davatchi F, Abdollahi BS, Mohyeddin M, et al. Mesenchymal stem cell therapy for knee osteoarthritis. Preliminary report of four patients. Int J Rheum Dis 2011;14(2):211–5.

96. Murphy JM, Fink DJ, Hunziker EB, et al. Stem cell therapy in a caprine model of osteoarthritis. Arthritis Rheum 2003;48(12):3464–74.

97. Wong KL, Lee KB, Tai BC, et al. Injectable cultured bone marrow-derived mesenchymal stem cells in varus knees with cartilage defects undergoing high tibial osteotomy: a prospective, randomized controlled clinical trial with 2 years' follow-up. Arthroscopy 2013;29(12):2020–8.

98. Kasemkijwattana C, Hongeng S, Kesprayura S, et al. Autologous bone marrow mesenchymal stem cells implantation for cartilage defects: two cases report. J Med Assoc Thai 2011;94(3): 395–400.

99. Wakitani S, Imoto K, Yamamoto T, et al. Human autologous culture expanded bone marrow mesenchymal cell transplantation for repair of cartilage defects in osteoarthritic knees. Osteoarthritis Cartilage 2002;10(3):199–206.

100. Wakitani S, Mitsuoka T, Nakamura N, et al. Autologous bone marrow stromal cell transplantation for repair of full-thickness articular cartilage defects in human patellae: two case reports. Cell Transplant 2004;13(5):595–600.

101. Kuroda R, Ishida K, Matsumoto T, et al. Treatment of a full-thickness articular cartilage defect in the femoral condyle of an athlete with autologous bone-marrow stromal cells. Osteoarthritis Cartilage 2007;15(2):226–31.

102. Haleem AM, Singergy AA, Sabry D, et al. The clinical use of human culture-expanded autologous bone marrow mesenchymal stem cells transplanted on platelet-rich fibrin glue in the treatment of articular cartilage defects: a pilot study and preliminary results. Cartilage 2010;1(4): 253–61.

103. Lee KB, Wang VT, Chan YH, et al. A novel, minimally-invasive technique of cartilage repair in the human knee using arthroscopic microfracture and injections of mesenchymal stem cells and hyaluronic acid–a prospective comparative study on safety and short-term efficacy. Ann Acad Med Singapore 2012;41(11):511–7.

104. Ishige I, Nagamura-Inoue T, Honda MJ, et al. Comparison of mesenchymal stem cells derived from arterial, venous, and Wharton's jelly explants of human umbilical cord. Int J Hematol 2009;90(2): 261–9.

105. McElreavey KD, Irvine AI, Ennis KT, et al. Isolation, culture and characterisation of fibroblast-like cells derived from the Wharton's jelly portion of human umbilical cord. Biochem Soc Trans 1991;19(1):29S.

106. Jeong SY, Kim DH, Ha J, et al. Thrombospondin-2 secreted by human umbilical cord blood-derived mesenchymal stem cells promotes chondrogenic differentiation. Stem Cells 2013;31(10):2136–48.

107. Zhang X, Hirai M, Cantero S, et al. Isolation and characterization of mesenchymal stem cells from human umbilical cord blood: reevaluation of critical factors for successful isolation and high ability to proliferate and differentiate to chondrocytes as compared to mesenchymal stem cells from bone marrow and adipose tissue. J Cell Biochem 2011;112(4):1206–18.

108. Nagamura-Inoue T, He H. Umbilical cord-derived mesenchymal stem cells: their advantages and potential clinical utility. World J Stem Cells 2014; 6(2):195–202.

109. Ha CW, Park YB, Chung JY, et al. Cartilage repair using composites of human umbilical cord blood-derived mesenchymal stem cells and hyaluronic acid hydrogel in a minipig model. Stem Cells Transl Med 2015;4(9):1044–51.

110. Park YB, Song M, Lee CH, et al. Cartilage repair by human umbilical cord blood-derived mesenchymal

stem cells with different hydrogels in a rat model. J Orthop Res 2015;33(11):1580–6.

111. Manferdini C, Maumus M, Gabusi E, et al. Adipose-derived mesenchymal stem cells exert anti-inflammatory effects on chondrocytes and synoviocytes from osteoarthritis patients through prostaglandin E2. Arthritis Rheum 2013;65(5):1271–81.

112. Wang YH, Wu JY, Chou PJ, et al. Characterization and evaluation of the differentiation ability of human adipose-derived stem cells growing in scaffold-free suspension culture. Cytotherapy 2014;16(4):485–95.

113. Mehlhorn AT, Niemeyer P, Kaschte K, et al. Differential effects of BMP-2 and TGF-beta1 on chondrogenic differentiation of adipose derived stem cells. Cell Prolif 2007;40(6):809–23.

114. Jo CH, Lee YG, Shin WH, et al. Intra-articular injection of mesenchymal stem cells for the treatment of osteoarthritis of the knee: a proof-of-concept clinical trial. Stem Cells 2014;32(5):1254–66.

115. Kim YS, Choi YJ, Suh DS, et al. Mesenchymal stem cell implantation in osteoarthritic knees: is fibrin glue effective as a scaffold? Am J Sports Med 2015;43(1):176–85.

116. Koh YG, Kwon OR, Kim YS, et al. Comparative outcomes of open-wedge high tibial osteotomy with platelet-rich plasma alone or in combination with mesenchymal stem cell treatment: a prospective study. Arthroscopy 2014;30(11):1453–60.

117. Koh YG, Choi YJ, Kwon OR, et al. Second-look arthroscopic evaluation of cartilage lesions after mesenchymal stem cell implantation in osteoarthritic knees. Am J Sports Med 2014;42(7):1628–37.

118. Koh YG, Choi YJ, Kwon SK, et al. Clinical results and second-look arthroscopic findings after treatment with adipose-derived stem cells for knee osteoarthritis. Knee Surg Sports Traumatol Arthrosc 2015;23(5):1308–16.

119. Chong PP, Selvaratnam L, Abbas AA, et al. Human peripheral blood derived mesenchymal stem cells demonstrate similar characteristics and chondrogenic differentiation potential to bone marrow derived mesenchymal stem cells. J Orthop Res 2012;30(4):634–42.

120. Saw KY, Anz A, Merican S, et al. Articular cartilage regeneration with autologous peripheral blood progenitor cells and hyaluronic acid after arthroscopic subchondral drilling: a report of 5 cases with histology. Arthroscopy 2011;27(4):493–506.

121. Saw KY, Anz A, Jee CS, et al. High tibial osteotomy in combination with chondrogenesis after stem cell therapy: a histologic report of 8 cases. Arthroscopy 2015;31(10):1909–20.

122. Fu WL, Ao YF, Ke XY, et al. Repair of large full-thickness cartilage defect by activating endogenous peripheral blood stem cells and autologous periosteum flap transplantation combined with patellofemoral realignment. Knee 2014;21(2):609–12.

123. Turajane T, Chaweewannakorn U, Larbpaiboonpong V, et al. Combination of intra-articular autologous activated peripheral blood stem cells with growth factor addition/preservation and hyaluronic acid in conjunction with arthroscopic microdrilling mesenchymal cell stimulation Improves quality of life and regenerates articular cartilage in early osteoarthritic knee disease. J Med Assoc Thai 2013;96(5):580–8.

124. Saw KY, Anz A, Siew-Yoke Jee C, et al. Articular cartilage regeneration with autologous peripheral blood stem cells versus hyaluronic acid: a randomized controlled trial. Arthroscopy 2013;29(4):684–94.

125. Orth P, Rey-Rico A, Venkatesan JK, et al. Current perspectives in stem cell research for knee cartilage repair. Stem Cells Cloning 2014;7:1–17.

126. Hatsushika D, Muneta T, Nakamura T, et al. Repetitive allogeneic intraarticular injections of synovial mesenchymal stem cells promote meniscus regeneration in a porcine massive meniscus defect model. Osteoarthritis Cartilage 2014;22(7):941–50.

127. Horie M, Sekiya I, Muneta T, et al. Intra-articular injected synovial stem cells differentiate into meniscal cells directly and promote meniscal regeneration without mobilization to distant organs in rat massive meniscal defect. Stem Cells 2009;27(4):878–87.

128. Mak J, Jablonski CL, Leonard CA, et al. Intra-articular injection of synovial mesenchymal stem cells improves cartilage repair in a mouse injury model. Sci Rep 2016;6:23076.

129. Sekiya I, Muneta T, Horie M, et al. Arthroscopic transplantation of synovial stem cells improves clinical outcomes in knees with cartilage defects. Clin Orthop Relat Res 2015;473(7):2316–26.

130. Akgun I, Unlu MC, Erdal OA, et al. Matrix-induced autologous mesenchymal stem cell implantation versus matrix-induced autologous chondrocyte implantation in the treatment of chondral defects of the knee: a 2-year randomized study. Arch Orthop Trauma Surg 2015;135(2):251–63.

131. Yoshiya S, Dhawan A. Cartilage repair techniques in the knee: stem cell therapies. Curr Rev Musculoskelet Med 2015;8(4):457–66.

132. Sanchez-Adams J, Athanasiou KA. Dermis isolated adult stem cells for cartilage tissue engineering. Biomaterials 2012;33(1):109–19.

133. Kalpakci KN, Brown WE, Hu JC, et al. Cartilage tissue engineering using dermis isolated adult stem cells: the use of hypoxia during expansion versus chondrogenic differentiation. PLoS One 2014;9(5):e98570.

134. Kuroda R, Usas A, Kubo S, et al. Cartilage repair using bone morphogenetic protein 4 and muscle-derived stem cells. Arthritis Rheum 2006;54(2):433–42.

135. Hsu SH, Huang TB, Cheng SJ, et al. Chondrogenesis from human placenta-derived mesenchymal stem cells in three-dimensional scaffolds for cartilage tissue engineering. Tissue Eng Part A 2011;17(11–12):1549–60.

136. Mizuno M, Kobayashi S, Takebe T, et al. Brief report: reconstruction of joint hyaline cartilage by autologous progenitor cells derived from ear elastic cartilage. Stem Cells 2014;32(3):816–21.

137. Li Q, Tang J, Wang R, et al. Comparing the chondrogenic potential in vivo of autogeneic mesenchymal stem cells derived from different tissues. Artif Cells Blood Substit Immobil Biotechnol 2011;39(1):31–8.

138. Hui JH, Li L, Teo YH, et al. Comparative study of the ability of mesenchymal stem cells derived from bone marrow, periosteum, and adipose tissue in treatment of partial growth arrest in rabbit. Tissue Eng 2005;11(5–6):904–12.

139. Nelson TJ, Martinez-Fernandez A, Terzic A. Induced pluripotent stem cells: developmental biology to regenerative medicine. Nat Rev Cardiol 2010;7(12):700–10.

140. Jopling C, Boue S, Izpisua Belmonte JC. Dedifferentiation, transdifferentiation and reprogramming: three routes to regeneration. Nat Rev Mol Cell Biol 2011;12(2):79–89.

141. Takahashi K, Yamanaka S. Induction of pluripotent stem cells from mouse embryonic and adult fibroblast cultures by defined factors. Cell 2006;126(4):663–76.

142. Koyanagi-Aoi M, Ohnuki M, Takahashi K, et al. Differentiation-defective phenotypes revealed by large-scale analyses of human pluripotent stem cells. Proc Natl Acad Sci U S A 2013;110(51):20569–74.

143. Takahashi K, Okita K, Nakagawa M, et al. Induction of pluripotent stem cells from fibroblast cultures. Nat Protoc 2007;2(12):3081–9.

144. Tsai SY, Bouwman BA, Ang YS, et al. Single transcription factor reprogramming of hair follicle dermal papilla cells to induced pluripotent stem cells. Stem Cells 2011;29(6):964–71.

145. Panopoulos AD, Ruiz S, Yi F, et al. Rapid and highly efficient generation of induced pluripotent stem cells from human umbilical vein endothelial cells. PLoS One 2011;6(5):e19743.

146. Aoi T, Yae K, Nakagawa M, et al. Generation of pluripotent stem cells from adult mouse liver and stomach cells. Science 2008;321(5889):699–702.

147. Utikal J, Maherali N, Kulalert W, et al. Sox2 is dispensable for the reprogramming of melanocytes and melanoma cells into induced pluripotent stem cells. J Cell Sci 2009;122(Pt 19):3502–10.

148. Sun N, Panetta NJ, Gupta DM, et al. Feeder-free derivation of induced pluripotent stem cells from adult human adipose stem cells. Proc Natl Acad Sci U S A 2009;106(37):15720–5.

149. Staerk J, Dawlaty MM, Gao Q, et al. Reprogramming of human peripheral blood cells to induced pluripotent stem cells. Cell Stem Cell 2010;7(1):20–4.

150. Loh YH, Hartung O, Li H, et al. Reprogramming of T cells from human peripheral blood. Cell Stem Cell 2010;7(1):15–9.

151. Zhao J, Jiang WJ, Sun C, et al. Induced pluripotent stem cells: origins, applications, and future perspectives. J Zhejiang Univ Sci B 2013;14(12):1059–69.

152. Uto S, Nishizawa S, Takasawa Y, et al. Bone and cartilage repair by transplantation of induced pluripotent stem cells in murine joint defect model. Biomed Res 2013;34(6):281–8.

153. Diekman BO, Christoforou N, Willard VP, et al. Cartilage tissue engineering using differentiated and purified induced pluripotent stem cells. Proc Natl Acad Sci U S A 2012;109(47):19172–7.

154. Ko JY, Kim KI, Park S, et al. In vitro chondrogenesis and in vivo repair of osteochondral defect with human induced pluripotent stem cells. Biomaterials 2014;35(11):3571–81.

155. Kim K, Doi A, Wen B, et al. Epigenetic memory in induced pluripotent stem cells. Nature 2010;467(7313):285–90.

156. Feng R, Desbordes SC, Xie H, et al. PU.1 and C/EBPalpha/beta convert fibroblasts into macrophage-like cells. Proc Natl Acad Sci U S A 2008;105(16):6057–62.

157. Caiazzo M, Dell'Anno MT, Dvoretskova E, et al. Direct generation of functional dopaminergic neurons from mouse and human fibroblasts. Nature 2011;476(7359):224–7.

158. Ring KL, Tong LM, Balestra ME, et al. Direct reprogramming of mouse and human fibroblasts into multipotent neural stem cells with a single factor. Cell Stem Cell 2012;11(1):100–9.

159. Vierbuchen T, Ostermeier A, Pang ZP, et al. Direct conversion of fibroblasts to functional neurons by defined factors. Nature 2010;463(7284):1035–41.

160. Fishman VS, Shnayder TA, Orishchenko KE, et al. Cell divisions are not essential for the direct conversion of fibroblasts into neuronal cells. Cell Cycle 2015;14(8):1188–96.

161. Sekiya S, Suzuki A. Direct conversion of mouse fibroblasts to hepatocyte-like cells by defined factors. Nature 2011;475(7356):390–3.

162. Szabo E, Rampalli S, Risueno RM, et al. Direct conversion of human fibroblasts to multilineage blood progenitors. Nature 2010;468(7323):521–6.

163. Efe JA, Hilcove S, Kim J, et al. Conversion of mouse fibroblasts into cardiomyocytes using a direct reprogramming strategy. Nat Cell Biol 2011;13(3):215–22.

164. Ieda M, Fu JD, Delgado-Olguin P, et al. Direct reprogramming of fibroblasts into functional cardiomyocytes by defined factors. Cell 2010;142(3): 375–86.

165. Hiramatsu K, Sasagawa S, Outani H, et al. Generation of hyaline cartilaginous tissue from mouse adult dermal fibroblast culture by defined factors. J Clin Invest 2011;121(2):640–57.

166. Outani H, Okada M, Hiramatsu K, et al. Induction of chondrogenic cells from dermal fibroblast culture by defined factors does not involve a pluripotent state. Biochem Biophys Res Commun 2011;411(3):607–12.

167. Ishii R, Kami D, Toyoda M, et al. Placenta to cartilage: direct conversion of human placenta to chondrocytes with transformation by defined factors. Mol Biol Cell 2012;23(18):3511–21.

Trauma

Bone Substitute Materials and Minimally Invasive Surgery
A Convergence of Fracture Treatment for Compromised Bone

Thomas A. Russell, MD[a],[*],[1], Gerard Insley, PhD[b]

KEYWORDS

- Calcium phosphates • Bone substitute materials (BSM) • Bone augmentation
- Calcium phosphate cements (CPC) • Internal fixation • Compromised bone
- Structural orthobiologic matrix (SOM) • Minimally Invasive Surgery (MIS)

KEY POINTS

- This article focuses key questions that can lead to the understanding and application of bone substitute materials (BSMs) that form a structural orthobiologic matrix within the metaphyseal components of the periarticular fracture.
- These 6 characteristics of BSMs are a rapid way for the surgeon to categorize the properties of BSMs and provide an algorithm for the selection of the optimal BSM.
- Advances in BSMs are synergistic with minimally invasive surgery (MIS) and have the potential for significant impact on orthopedic patients' health and socioeconomic viability after injury.
- Calcium phosphate cements in combination with MIS techniques and implants can enhance rehabilitation and recovery and lead to the realization of the vision of immediate postoperative load bearing of our patients with periarticular fracture.

INTRODUCTION

The past 35 years have been unprecedented as a time of innovation in orthopedic surgery with regard to surgical techniques, procedures, and metal alloy biomaterial fabrication with patients benefitting from reduced deformity, earlier mobilization, and decreased permanent disability after skeletal injury and disease.

Minimally invasive surgery (MIS) allows for safe insertion of sophisticated implants while causing the least possible trauma to the soft tissue environment of injury and to patients. MIS is still evolving through advances in incision design, surgical implants and instruments with the aid of a wide variety of imaging technologies (intraoperative computed tomographic scanning

Conflicts of Interest: T.A. Russell holds intellectual property contracts with Smith & Nephew, Memphis, TN and Zimmer Biomet, Warsaw, IN and is an inventor of N-Force systems. He is a consultant for Zimmer Biomet in Trauma and Biomaterials. G. Insley, PhD is Chief Science Officer for CelgenTek Innovations Corporation (CIC).
[a] Department of Orthopedic Surgery, Campbell Clinic, University of Tennessee Center for the Health Sciences, University of Tennessee, 1211 Union Ave, Memphis, TN 38104, USA; [b] Celgen Tek, Western Business Park, Shannon, Co. Clare, Ireland
[1] 240 LaGrange Creek Drive, Eads, TN 38028, USA.
* Corresponding author.
E-mail address: tarmd100@gmail.com

Orthop Clin N Am 48 (2017) 289–300
http://dx.doi.org/10.1016/j.ocl.2017.03.003
0030-5898/17/© 2017 Elsevier Inc. All rights reserved.

and MRI) as well as the more recent development of computer-assisted technology.[1]

When bone is damaged by crush or loss of tissue, surgical stabilization and subsequent bone regeneration may be impossible without the addition of materials to address the bone defect. Bone substitute materials (BSMs) are evolving in parallel with advances in MIS to meet patients' demands for more rapid recovery from musculoskeletal injury permitting earlier weight bearing, leading to earlier return to work and recreation.

This article focuses on the understanding and application of BSM and particularly the newer calcium phosphate materials that can form a structural orthobiologic matrix within the metaphyseal components of the periarticular fracture. Primarily, there are 6 characteristics of BSMs that can be used as a guide for the proper selection and application of the optimal BSM type for periarticular fracture repair, and these are discussed in detail.

BONE

Bones comprising the skeletal system are dynamic organs with mineral, cellular, molecular, and vascular components. Bone is a "fiber-reinforced composite of a biological origin, in which nanometer-sized hard inclusions are embedded into a soft protein matrix."[2] Bone is produced by specialized interacting cells known as a bone metabolic unit, which consist of osteoclasts, osteoblasts, and osteocytes, working together to form bone structural units (BSUs). These BSUs are the building blocks of the bone lamellae and subsequent composites of cortical and cancellous bone that form the specific skeletal bone. These units have a finite life span with a range of 3 to 20 years depending on the metabolic requirements of the host and structural demands on the bone. During fracture healing, woven bone is produced initially and is converted to the more resilient lamellar bone by a process known as bone remodeling. Normal bone remodeling is a coordinated cyclic process of bone resorption (osteoclasts) and bone formation (osteoblasts). The main functions of bone remodeling are reshaping and replacement of bone during growth and following injury and trauma; preserving bone strength by removing old (micro) damaged bone and replacing it with newer mechanically stronger bone; and involvement in calcium and phosphate homeostasis. Along with remodeling, bone has the capacity of regeneration, which is a tightly regulated process of bone formation evidenced in fracture healing and is associated with continuous remodeling throughout adult life.[3] Bone's capability for regeneration is the key to the utility of bioavailable calcium phosphate cements (CPCs) in critical size defects and reinforcement/augmentation of internal fixation in compromised bone.

Bone has several unique attributes, including its physical properties of flexible rigidity, optimal strength to weight ratio, ability for self-repair through osteogenesis after injury, and contribution to the metabolic stability of the body as its primary reserve for vital minerals, including calcium, phosphate, magnesium, sodium, and carbonate. Each bone is individually structured for its respective contribution to mobility, anchorage and protection of the soft tissues, and physical interaction with a person's environment. When bone is damaged by injury or disease, such that its' normal repair/regeneration cycle is compromised, augmentation with synthetic BSMs may assist in prevention of deformity and nonunion (in conjunction with modern surgical implants and techniques).

DIAMOND CONCEPT

As already stated, bone possesses a considerable capacity for regeneration following trauma. A complex pathway of both physiologic and biomechanical interactions are required in order for fracture healing to occur. These processes can be illustrated using the Diamond Concept. The Diamond Concept of fracture healing relates the interaction of osteogenic cells, osteoinductive signals, and osteoconductive scaffolds with surgical reconstruction with implants in achieving bone repair (Fig. 1). The Diamond

Augmentation Diamond Concept

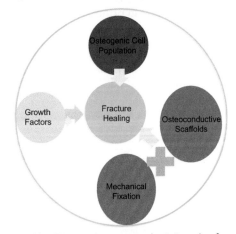

Fig. 1. The Diamond concept, depicting the factors effecting fracture healing. (*Adapted from* Giannoudis PV, Einhorn TA, Marsh D. Fracture healing: the diamond concept. Injury 2007;38 Suppl 4:S5; with permission.)

concept of fracture repair groups the components required for successful fracture healing.[4] This article focuses on one particular aspect of the Diamond concept, the osteoconductive scaffold group.

THE OSTEOCONDUCTIVE GROUP

BSMs represent the osteoconductive component of the Diamond concept paradigm and at this time should not be considered osteoinductive or cell delivery systems (new developments to attain these attributes are in the research arena). Although they lack the osteoinductive/osteogenic properties, they promote migration, proliferation, and differentiation of bone cells for bone regeneration. As such, they provide structural material, although not necessarily structure to the fracture site. Optimally, they act as matrix materials for the ingrowth of new bone while minimizing dead space and the possibility of connective tissue replacement of the bone defect with scar formation.

BSMs are usually synthetic in that they are produced from sintering chemically formed compounds or through precipitation wet chemical route. As these synthetic BSMs are chemically created, their physical properties are easily altered and reproduced. The microstructure of the synthetic BSMs can be optimized to mimic human cancellous bone by adjusting the chemical formulations as well as optimizing its osteoconductive properties.[5,6] Within the United States, the Food and Drug Administration (FDA) has limited the regulatory clearance of most of these synthetic BSMs to being used when the void is minor or non–load bearing when used in isolation. In Europe, regulatory clearances have permitted third-generation premix CPCs and augmented fixation devices to be widely available.

There are several synthetic BSMs currently available, including hydroxyapatite (HA), tricalcium phosphate (TCP), CPCs, and glass ceramics.[7] HA is similar to the mineral component of natural bone, is a naturally occurring mineral form of calcium apatite, and is considered extremely biocompatible. Synthetic HAs in their many forms are one of the most common BSMs used.[8] TCP, another common compound of bone, acts efficiently as an osteoconductive scaffold and is more soluble and less crystalline than HA allowing it to be more readily resorbed.[9] TCP exists in 2 forms: alpha (α) and beta (β) TCP. α-TCP is more soluble than β-TCP and resorbs faster in vivo.[9]

Biphasic calcium phosphates are produced by combinations of calcium phosphates, such as HA and TCP. Its rate of resorption depends on the amount of each used to generate the BSM.

Calcium sulfates are also often used as a BSM. Calcium sulfates can dissolve and resorb extremely quickly, usually within a period of weeks, which renders it unsuitable for instances whereby long-term scaffolding is required for growth.

Longer-acting osteoconductive BSMs address the clinical problems of insufficient bone quality or quantity. In intraarticular fractures, proper placement of flowable CPCs may retard the influx of synovial fluid, which contains antiangiogenic factors that may compromise revascularization of the fracture site. However, there are critical factors the orthopedic surgeon needs to be aware of to ensure safe and effective use of these materials. Common clinical concerns include

1. Infection/contamination at the injury site
2. Neoplasm/cystic processes within Osteolytic voids at the injury site
3. The extent of surgically induced defects from osteotomies and arthroplasty as to gross structural stability
4. Reconstruction of open fractures with bone extrusion and loss
5. Analysis of impaction loss with periarticular metaphyseal of the intraarticular components of cartilage and soft tissues combined with the cancellous and cortical bone loss
6. Osteopenia compromising bone implant anchorage

IMPLANT STABILIZATION AND AUGMENTATION: POLYMETHYL METHACRYLATE VERSUS BONE SUBSTITUTE MATERIALS

The initial concepts of implant stabilization at the interface of the bone implant junction were developed for total joint arthroplasty by Charnley in 1958.[10] Since then there has been an abundance of material specifically developed for implant stabilization and augmentation. For a surgeon, the selection of which material to use for an indication, the method to prepare it, and how to place it in the optimal position are critical factors in whether to choose products composed of polymethyl methacrylate (PMMA), BSMs, or other augmentation materials. **Fig. 2** illustrates and compares the differences between bone cement (PMMA) and CPCs.

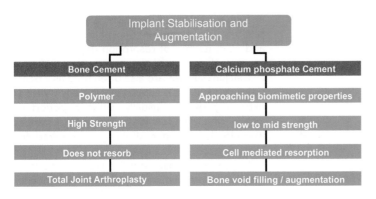

Fig. 2. Implant stabilization and augmentation. This figure illustrates and compares the differences between bone cement (products composed of PMMA) and CPCs.

Bone cement or PMMA is a biostable polymer of carbon $(C_5O_2H_8)_n$, also known as acrylic, that undergoes polymerization when activated as opposed to the crystallization process of the calcium orthophosphate cements and has no potential for remodeling. Harrington and Johnston[11] and Bartucci and colleagues[12] reported the use of PMMA in fracture care in osteoporotic fractures, but initial results were compromised by the inhibition of fracture healing. Additionally, difficulties with extravasation and requisite high-pressure injection methods discouraged widespread use in nonpathologic fractures.[11,12]

CHARACTERISTICS OF BONE SUBSTITUTE MATERIAL

Synthetic BSMs are complex molecules and composites unlike any other implants surgeons use with regard to function, preparation, handling, and placement. For a surgeon to use these materials in surgery, the selection of which material to be used and how to prepare it and place it in the optimal position are as critical as knowing what size and type of implant (ie, plate) as well as the number and location of screws to use. For example, in younger patients, the option of complete biological conversion to new bone is most desirable, whereas, in older patients, a longer stable mechanical structure may be desirable because of the impaired osteogenic potential in the older host. In cases of bacterial contamination, calcium sulfates may be used alone or in combination with antibiotics at the surgeons' discretion to help control contamination as they dissolve with no residual material. CPCs should not be used in contaminated wounds as they may become foci for bacterial biofilm production.

The analysis to determine the optimal application of a BSM requires an understanding of the 6 characteristics. These 6 characteristics of BSMs can be divided into 2 pillars:

1. The biochemistry of BSMs
2. The surgical application of BSMs (Table 1)

The biochemistry pillar encompasses molecular formulae, morphology, and metabolism; the surgical application pillar includes the mechanical properties, material preparation, and material placement, all of which are discussed in detail later.

BIOCHEMISTRY: PILLAR I

Biochemistry looks at structure, function, and interaction of biological macromolecules within a host organism. In this case, it is BSMs' structure and function as a bone remodeler that is critical. In examining the molecular formula, morphology, and porosity of BSMs, a greater analysis can be made as to how these BSMs will function in their role as bone remodelers within the body and the properties they will contribute to the material

Table 1 The 6 characteristics of bone substitute materials	
Biochemistry	**Surgical Application**
Molecular formulae	Material preparation
Morphology	Mechanical properties
Metabolism	Material placement

The characteristics of BSMs are shown here divided into 2 pillars: the biochemistry pillar encompassing molecular formulae, morphology, and metabolism and the surgical application pillar containing the mechanical properties, material preparation, and material placement.

used by the surgeon. Investigating BSMs' metabolism reveals the conversion of their biological signals into downstream process and applications. This information is a key piece of information the surgeon requires when determining what material to use, particularly in fracture healing processes.

Molecular Formulae

The molecular formulae of the BSM is most commonly one of 3 types:

- A combination of calcium sulfate and granular hydroxyapatite
- A calcium sulfate
- Calcium phosphate composite

The molecular formulae of human bone mineral is expressed as $Ca1_{0-x}(M)_x(PO4)_{6-x}(HPO4, CO3)_x(OH)_{2-x}$ and is different from granular HA as it is populated with metal ions, most commonly magnesium and carbonate.[8]

The calcium sulfates, $CaSO_4$, are simple ionic salts. These materials rapidly dissolve in water releasing calcium ions and produce a pH acidic shift due to the sulfate ions combining with hydrogen. Therefore, calcium sulfate materials do not remodel through cell-mediated processes rather they dissolve readily independent of bone ingrowth or repair.

Calcium phosphates are covalently bound molecules and are more stable in an aqueous environment. They vary from simple $Ca_3(HPO_4)$ molecules to complex biomimetic molecular forms very similar to human bone mineral.

Silicates may be added to calcium phosphates but their effect on bone healing has been a matter of some debate.[13] Early work done by Carlisle[14] suggests that silicon is present during new bone formation in the early stages of biomineralization but it decreases to a negligible amount as the final physiologic HA is formed. This work has led researchers to consider silicon as an additive to HA to induce a faster remodeling response. In more recent work, Patel and colleagues[15] advocated the use of silicon substitute TCP; their early preclinical work demonstrated an increase in the speed and quality of the bone repair process. The mode of action for the silicon substituted HA materials as proposed by Pietak and colleagues[16] show that the presence of the ion modifies the surface chemistry of the material through modification of the surface microstructure giving increased solubility rates rather than any metabolic cell-based interaction. Despite the preclinical research and the many claims made for silicon substituted biomaterials' increased efficacy, there is no substantial clinical evidence

showing an increased healing that would be relevant to a surgeon.[17]

The molecular formulae of these materials are important because as advanced calcium phosphates' molecular formulae more closely resemble that of human bone mineral, then the biocompatible bone matrix substitute materials formed are capable of maintaining structure until the required remodeling occurs by bone metabolic units.

Morphology

The term *morphology* simply means the particular shape, form, or structure of the material. In the case of BSMs, the form and shape can include flowing self-setting cements, irregular granules, regular-shape blocks (wedges, discs, and so forth), and putties. In the case of augmenting fractures in MIS surgery, the most advantageous form is the flowable self-setting CPCs. These materials have the unique ability to be a flowing viscous liquid allowing surgical delivery and filling of a bone void through a small entry hole in the bone. Once in place, the materials then undergo a setting process and move from a liquid phase through a paste phase to finally set as a solid phase with enough mechanical strength to maintain volume and remain where placed.

Flowing calcium phosphate materials are available with enhancements provided by additives to induce pore formation of size and interconnectivity to encourage enhanced surface area and revascularization capability after crystallization is completed.[18] These flowing CPCs are generally non-Newtonian fluidic materials with atypical fluid behavior when compared with water (a Newtonian material) in that their viscosity and ability to flow are time dependent and inversely related to insertion pressure and the reciprocal shear that force induces.[19] Counterintuitively, pushing harder on an injection device for a non-Newtonian CPC will reduce its capability to flow; if a critical insertion force is exceeded, the CPC will phase separate (separation of the hydration fluid and the powder) inactivating the CPC and preventing further flow.

With MIS techniques, the bone defect is closed before insertion of the BSM by the fracture reduction. The BSM must be contained within the bone for optimal function and metabolism. When the surgeon tries to inject the BSM with a needle or cannula, a pressure gradient inside the closed defect develops from residual blood and debris within the fracture (Venturi effect of pressure equalization with noncompressible fluids in closed chambers). This pressure gradient results in extrusion of the material at the entry site and incomplete fill (Fig. 3). Larger cannulas may be used,

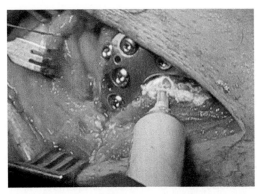

Fig. 3. Extrusion of the material at the entry site. Venturi effect (a pressure gradient develops within the closed defect due to the buildup of blood and debris within the fracture) results in the extrusion of the material at the entry site and causes an incomplete fill of the void.

but the material may leak out into the soft tissues from the holes created. A secondary problem may be extrusion of the BSM into the joint or out of the fracture zone in comminuted fractures when one tries to increase the pressure of injection. This extrusion may be the primary reason for slow adoption of BSM in the past despite the level of evidence for its superiority over cancellous autograph and allograft bone tissue with regard to structural stability of the articular reduction.

New developments in CPC have combined calcium phosphates with surfactants, such as carboxymethylcellulose and lipids, to change the flow characteristics of the non-Newtonian CPCs. In experimental and cadaveric femoral studies, CPCs could be differentiated by their flow characteristics and their intrusion or lack of intrusion into trabecular bone.[20,21] These enhanced CPCs allow better control of material delivery into the reduced fracture site.

The next important morphologic attribute is porosity of the material. Porosity is essentially the amount of void space present in the final material and is usually shown as a percentage of the total implant volume. Typically, material porosity is described as either macroporosity (>50 μm) or microporosity (<10 μm) and also the level in percent of how interconnected the pores are. In the self-setting CPCs, most of the porosity is in the microporosity range and is highly interconnected. Interconnected microporosity allows proliferation and diffusion of nutrients throughout the BSM, thus, influencing the speed of bone remodeling.

Therefore, the morphology of the synthetic BSMs is an important property to keep in mind when a surgeon is planning MIS fracture management. The morphology effects how easily

the surgeon can deliver and place the material (flowable) and its surface area available for cell-mediated resorption (porosity).

Metabolism

The third characteristic is metabolism of the BSM and may be one of the most important branch points in decision-making. When the authors consider bone augmentation, they expect an interaction with the augmentation biomaterial with the host bone and body. This interaction can be of 4 types: (1) biostable: no host reaction and no incorporation; (2) biodegradation with dissolution of the material through hydrolysis (PLA [Polylactic Acid]- and PGA [Polyglycolic Acid]-type polymers); (3) biodegradation by salt dissolution (calcium sulfates); (4) biodegradation by cell-mediated resorption with biomaterial resorption and osteogenesis connecting the new bone to the adjacent bone. This type of remodeling may be partial or complete depending on the reactivity of the material, its porosity, and pore characteristics (size and interconnectivity).

In choosing a BSM, the surgeon needs to think about how the material is going to interact with the bone during the fracture healing process and indeed beyond. In the case of MIS fracture management, the CPCs have the advantage of being osteoconductive and remodel through interaction directly with the bone metabolic units leading to a predictable outcome that works with the body's fracture healing processes.

SURGICAL APPLICATION: PILLAR II

The next 3 Ms in pillar II concern the structural properties of the BSM, which may be either nonexistent or equivalent to bone itself when fully cured in its final crystalline state; the difficulty and precision required in the intraoperative preparation of the materials; and the placement into the proper anatomic location within the bone and adjacent to the surgical implants for fracture stabilization.

Mechanical/Material Properties

This fourth characteristic relates to BSM mechanical properties. Compressive strength, tensile strength, and flow characteristics are material properties. Calcium sulfates have essentially no long-term structural support capability because of their salt dissolution. Calcium phosphates have variable compressive strengths of 4 MPa to 60 MPa, based on the manufacturer's design. They are stronger in compression than tension and are brittle in isolation. The human Cancellous metaphyseal bone averages 8 to 12 MPa of compressive stiffness but gains its strength from the structural properties of gradient deposition of bone and overlap of lamellae, which yields either cortical or cancellous bone architecture, depending on the density of the lamellae. BSM may also be optimally placed to improve its overall mechanical support by integrating it within the cancellous networks. Cortical replacement by synthetic BSM in diaphyseal fractures is not yet possible, but 3-dimensional printing developments may yield such materials in the near future.

Therefore, the mechanical properties of BSMs tend to be in the region of cancellous bone and should not be considered as materials that can bear physiologic loads in the body independently. BSMs are typically designed to be cohesive enough to withstand intraoperative delivery and placement by the surgeon and then are strong enough to maintain volume and, where necessary, augment fracture hardware, such as bone screws.

Material Preparation

Material preparation is the fifth characteristic of self-hardening BSM, as granular or block BSMs do not require mixing. Typically, the Self-hardening BSM is supplied as a sterile kit containing the calcium sulfate, calcium phosphate or combination powder with the appropriate mixing/injection equipment. At the point of care, the constituents of the BSM are combined, mixed homogenously, and delivered by the surgeon. The setting reaction begins immediately; depending on the formulation, over a period of time the BSM will transform into a biomaterial that is apatite HA, calcium-deficient HA, or brushite (DCPD) in nature, whereas the calcium sulfates will harden as a salt that is rapidly hydrolyzed. Even if the calcium sulfate is mixed with a HA particulate dispersion, no structural matrix will form. The setting reaction will either be hydrolytic or acid-base in nature, again depending on the original formulation.[22,23] In a hydrolytic reaction forming apatite cement, at least one component of the CPC should be an aqueous solution in order to initiate the cement setting reactions after mixing the components.

There is a history of studies as far back as the 1920s using calcium phosphates in the repair of bone defects.[24–26] Since that time calcium phosphate has evolved through 3 generations of development.

First-generation calcium phosphates were granular calcium phosphate materials. They were generally HA or β-TCP in nature and were well established having both biocompatible and osteoconductive properties. β-TCP demonstrated greater solubility in physiologic environments than HA.[27,28] In 1951 Ray and Ward[26] demonstrated that HA was replaced by new bone, but these first-generation materials were not as effective as autogenous bone grafts in repairing the defects. Clinically, granular particular BSMs are highly useful either alone or in combination with tissue transfer components of whole graft, demineralized bone matrix, and processed allograft bone or used as osteoconductive fillers in polymeric tissue scaffolds.[25] One of the main problems with these materials lies in the fact that all of them had issues with delivery and placement. Granules that are in a vial are not useful to a surgeon when he or she has to fill an osteolytic void in the upper part of the acetabulum or indeed when delivery through a 4-mm drill hole is required, as in the case frequently with MIS.

In an attempt to address these shortcomings, a new type of self-hardening cement consisting primarily of calcium phosphate and that formed HA as a product when hardened was developed by Brown and Chow[29,30] in the early 1980s.

These second-generation BSMs form mostly apatite products, but there are some that form brushite (DCPD). However, all have similar in vivo properties despite the differences in their starting material and have largely been the mainstay of BSMs currently used in fracture surgery today. The primary advantage of the second-generation CPCs is that they are cohesive and moldable but poorly injectable, which is of crucial importance to surgeons. This generation of BSM was designed for open reduction procedures whereby the defect was openly explored and surgically placed before definitive fracture reduction and definitive fixation. Currently this generation of CPCs is commonly presented in a powder and liquid form that requires manual mixing and multiple preparation steps before injecting; they also have limited or no stop-start inject ability as well as varying working and set times. They have been difficult to place and retain in the optimal position at the surgical site, and MIS techniques have compounded these difficulties with these materials. Stop-start ability is the ability to stop and restart the BSM activation during surgery to permit extended working time and multiple injection sites with the same material package and is currently available commercially in Europe.

Flowable BSMs offer the potential of reinforcement and augmentation of the surgical implant fixation into the bone in the metaphyseal regions of implant attachment and thereby prevent displacement of fracture fragments. There is now level 1 to 3 evidence of superiority of self-hardening BSMs in the prevention of subarticular collapse compared with autograft or allograft bone tissue transfer (grafting) in the tibial plateau, calcaneus, and acetabular fractures and reduced implant failure when used to reinforce screw fixation.[31–35]

There is a critical ratio of powder to liquid with CPC, which is under control of the surgeon intraoperatively. Insufficient hydration leaves the mixture too solid to inject, and too much hydration prevents the nucleation/crystallization reaction from developing into a solid matrix. Intraoperative mixing and compounding, therefore, require precision and compliance with the manufacturer's recommendations. Time of workability depends on the flow phase of the material, which depends on its rate of viscosity increase with time, as a non-Newtonian fluid. As discussed, excessive insertion force or inadequate powder/liquid ratios will decrease the working time. Materials are calibrated for fast setting (1–3 minutes) or slow setting (6 minutes to 30 minutes) depending on the manufacturer's formulation. Knowledge of the manufacturers design specifications is critical to success. Manual syringe or assisted injection devices are matched with the material from the manufacturer and require preoperative education to the nursing team and surgeon to insure proper use during surgery (**Fig. 4**).

These disadvantages have necessitated new research and development, which have given rise to third-generation CPCs. To enhance clinical usefulness, the surgeon would prefer a premixed cement that can be placed directly in the defect within a prescribed time. These next-generation products have 4 common design criteria:

1. The cement must have minimal or no preparation steps.
2. It must be directly implantable.
3. It must be capable of extended shelf life for hospital inventory management.

4. There must be surgeon-controlled working and setting times.

Third-generation CPCs are similar to second-generation CPCs in that they are injectable and form mostly apatite products with a few forming DCPD products.[36] But this is where the similarities end. These new-generation CPCs are premixed, are ready to inject, and are now a point-and-shoot technology. These premixed formulations can be supplied as dual-paste premix formulations, with one of the pastes being aqueous (to initiate the setting reaction) and the other being nonaqueous (containing the calcium phosphate). Unlike second-generation CPCs, third-generation technology has stop-start inject ability up to about 2 hours, giving the surgeon control of the reaction time. Third-generation BSMs harden more uniformly and have controlled viscosity and controlled setting times, making them more compatible with augmentation fixation technology.

Premixed CPCs are a new development to surgical efficiency to minimize mixing errors and shorten the surgical time for the BSM application. Premixed CPCs are formulated to stabilize the various calcium phosphates and necessary reactants in pastelike components. For premixed injectable CPCs, water-immiscible carrier liquids are often used for the preparation and stabilization of the calcium phosphate component. As a result, the setting reaction of the cement takes place after definitive substitution of the carrier liquid in the CPC paste with the aqueous solution, where both liquids are separated by a sharp interface (**Fig. 5**). During this reaction, 3 stages occur:

1. Dissolution of the reactants
2. Nucleation of the new HA phase
3. Crystal growth[37]

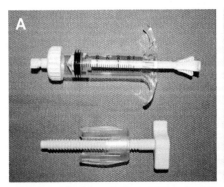
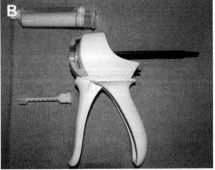

Fig. 4. (*A*) Mixing and insertion devices. (*B*) Premix delivery system. (*A*) A mixing preparation system that requires preoperative education of the nursing team and surgeon to insure proper use during surgery. (*B*) A new premix delivery system that is ready to inject and is now point-and-shoot technology.

1. CPC paste suspended in water immiscible liquid

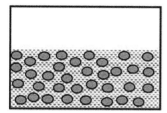

2. Introduction of water and extraction of immiscible liquid from the CPC paste

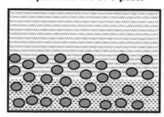

3. Definitive substitution of the carrier liquid in the CPC paste with water

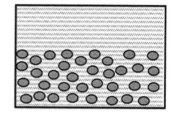

4. Dissolution and precipitation process

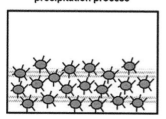

5. Final HA crystals

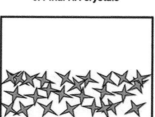

Fig. 5. The setting reaction of HA forming CPC paste following the introduction of aqueous solution (water).

Throughout the dissolution process, the raw powders in the formulation release calcium and phosphate ions, thereby producing a supersaturation in the solution. When the ionic concentration reaches a critical value, nucleation of the new phase takes place, thus, surrounding the powder particles. After this, the new phase continues to develop as the dissolution of the reagents occurs over time. Over the first few hours the setting process is governed by the dissolution kinetics of the raw materials; however, once the reactants are completely surrounded by the new phase, the setting process is governed by diffusion throughout the new phase.[22,36] Depending on formulation, complete setting of the cement is normally concluded between 24 and 72 hours.

Therefore, material preparation is a critical factor to consider for surgeons, especially when they are faced with the many BSMs on the market. Clearly the third-generation materials that offer minimal preparation steps and are literally point and shoot out of the pack with the added benefit of the ability to stop and start the delivery are destined to be the standard for osteoconductive BSM.

MATERIAL PLACEMENT

Finally, material placement of the CPC is the sixth characteristic: Where should the CPC implant be placed? This placement depends on the requirements for the BSM. If the defect is a simple void, such as a cyst or biopsy site, a hole is drilled and the appropriate cannula for BSM delivery is inserted into the defect. A vent hole or second cannula should be drilled to ensure a complete fill. If the defect is critically adjacent to subchondral fragments, it must be filled with adequate volume directly beneath the articular fracture fragments.[38]

AUGMENTATION OPTIONS FOR OSTEOPENIC OR OSTEOPOROTIC BONE

When augmenting a defect with poor bone quality from osteopenia or fracture comminution there are 3 options available:

1. Place the CPC into a predrilled hole in the bone and then place the screw into the drilled hole. In practice, this is problematic

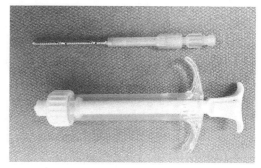

Fig. 6. N-Force Fixation system. The first FDA-cleared fracture implant (a fenestrated screw) optimized for hydraulic flow of CPC into a defect in cancellous bone. (Zimmer Biomet, Warsaw, IN)

because in this case the surgeon is filling a space that is full of body fluid and the cement has to displace this fluid first in order to effectively fill the predrilled hole. If there is no vent in place, often the cement will extrude back out the hole and not fill effectively.

2. Insert the CPC and let it harden, and then drill through the material and insert the screw. This option is problematic, as it may destroy the structural integrity of the CPC matrix.

3. Execute CPC delivery through the fracture fixation device. This type of placement optimizes the material around the designated area of the implant. There are 2 techniques for CPC delivery through the fixation implant:

   a. *Point augmentation* whereby the implant is cannulated with distal predesigned fenestrations: A second cannula is inserted

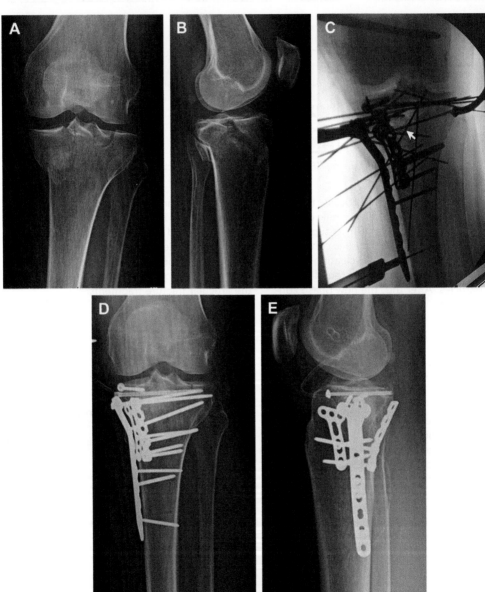

Fig. 7. (A) Preoperative anteroposterior radiograph demonstrating Schatzker 4 tibial plateau fracture. (B) Preoperative lateral radiograph. (C) Intraoperative reduction with central defect. (Arrow denotes residual defect after skeletal repair) (D) Postoperative anteroposterior radiograph with N-Force augmentation and definitive plate fixation. (E) Postoperative lateral radiograph with N-Force augmentation and definitive plate fixation. (*Courtesy of* G.S. Marecek, MD, Los Angeles, CA.)

up into the device to the level of the fenestrations, and the BSM material can be inserted into the specified area of bone. Limited amounts of material are possible with this technique. Regulatory clearances for this technique are available in Europe and the United States.

  b. *Near cortical circumferential augmentation*: This augmentation is a new development of a fenestrated screw or intraosseous implant optimized for hydraulic flow of CPC to fill the defective cancellous bone architecture but also to permit augmentation of the cortex at the implant insertion site. This technique serves to reinforce the structural stability of the implant along its length and not just at one location. The N-Force Fixation System (Zimmer Biomet, Warsaw, IN) was the first FDA-cleared fracture implant with this ability (**Fig. 6**) and is available in Europe and the United States. **Fig. 7** demonstrates a case using this technology.

SUMMARY

There are numerous clinical benefits in combining the new technologies of BSMs with those of MIS, especially those that meet the patients' demands for more rapid recovery from earlier weight bearing and social-economic factors, such as return to work and recreation. The combination of BSM and MIS technologies may also lead to an improvement in the quality of life by reducing the instances of revision surgery.

MIS minimizes the collateral damage from surgical intervention compared with open extensile procedures, which tend to compromise the adjacent soft tissue structures. The bone itself benefits from MIS technique by the preservation of the vascular environment of the bone outside of the zone of injury. MIS techniques have been optimized for weight-bearing diaphyseal fractures with interlocking closed-section nailing techniques in the femur and tibia. Periarticular fractures have been more challenging because of the transitional nature of the cortical tubular diaphysis to the metaphyseal cancellous network supporting the articular cartilage. MIS implants and techniques have resulted in lowered implant loss of reduction but have required new skills, instruments, implants, and intraoperative monitoring of the injury site with image intensification radiography, instead of direct optical visualization and tactile analysis of the fracture defect to obtain reduction and place fixation. The quantity and quality of bone loss may be difficult to evaluate with MIS

techniques and may compromise the stability of surgical implants resulting in subsequent loss of reduction, deformity, and morbidity.

Advances in BSM are synergistic with MIS and have the potential for significant impact on orthopedic patients' health and socioeconomic viability after injury. The ability to regain early functional ambulation after tibial and femoral diaphyseal fractures with interlocking intramedullary nailing and internal fixation of spinal injury is proof of the feasibility to set the same goals for patients with periarticular fractures.

BSM especially CPCs in combination with MIS techniques, including implants with CPC delivery capability, are catching up with the rapid development of locking plate technology and interlocking intramedullary nail techniques. There is a real opportunity for the synergy of these technologies to attain the next level of enhanced rehabilitation and recovery and realize the vision of immediate postoperative load bearing of patients with periarticular fractures.

ACKNOWLEDGMENTS

The authors appreciate the assistance of Regina O'Sullivan PhD, Kieran Murray PhD, and Dr Geoff Marecek for their contributions to this article.

REFERENCES

1. Yeung SH. Minimally invasive surgery in orthopaedics. Small is beautiful? Hong Kong Med J 2008; 14(4):303–7.
2. Ji B, Gao H. Elastic properties of nanocomposite structure of bone. Composites Sci Technology 2006;66(9):1212–8.
3. Dimitriou R, Jones E, McGonagle D, et al. Bone regeneration: current concepts and future directions. BMC Med 2011;9:66.
4. Giannoudis PV, Einhorn TA, Marsh D. Fracture healing: the diamond concept. Injury 2007; 38(Suppl 4):S3–6.
5. Resnick DK. Vitoss bone substitute. Neurosurgery 2002;50(5):1162–4.
6. Boschetti F, Tomei AA, Turri S, et al. Design, fabrication, and characterization of a composite scaffold for bone tissue engineering. Int J Artif Organs 2008;31(8):697–707.
7. Giannoudis PV, Dinopoulos H, Tsiridis E. Bone substitutes: an update. Injury 2005;36(Suppl 3):S20–7.
8. LeGeros RZ. Properties of osteoconductive biomaterials: calcium phosphates. Clin Orthop Relat Res 2002;(395):81–98.
9. Gazdag AR, Lane JM, Glaser D, et al. Alternatives to autogenous bone graft: efficacy and indications. J Am Acad Orthop Surg 1995;3(1):1–8.

10. Fenton P, Rampurada A, Qureshi F. Bone Cement, its History, its Properties and Developments in its Use. USM Orthopaedic for Postgraduate: a Blog dedicated to orthopaedic residents. 2009. Available at: http://www.usmorthopaedic.wordpress.com/2009/08/24. Accessed August 24, 2009.

11. Bartucci EJ, Gonzalez MH, Cooperman DR, et al. The effect of adjunctive methyl methacrylate on failures of fixation and function in patients with intertrochanteric fractures and osteoporosis. J Bone Joint Surg Am 1985;67(7):1094–107.

12. Harrington KD, Johnston JO. The management of comminuted unstable intertrochanteric fractures. J Bone Joint Surg Am 1973;55(7):1367–76.

13. Bohner M. Silicon-substituted calcium phosphates - a critical view. Biomaterials 2009;30(32):6403–6.

14. Carlisle EM. Silicon: a possible factor in bone calcification. Science 1970;167(3916):279–80.

15. Patel N, Brooks RA, Clarke MT, et al. In vivo assessment of hydroxyapatite and silicate-substituted hydroxyapatite granules using an ovine defect model. J Mater Sci Mater Med 2005;16(5):429–40.

16. Pietak AM, Reid JW, Stott MJ, et al. Silicon substitution in the calcium phosphate bioceramics. Biomaterials 2007;28(28):4023–32.

17. Kurien T, Pearson RG, Scammell BE. Bone graft substitutes currently available in orthopaedic practice: the evidence for their use. Bone Joint J 2013; 95B(5):583–97.

18. Bercier A, Gonçalves S, Lignon O, et al. Calcium phosphate bone cements including sugar surfactants: part one—porosity, setting times and compressive strength. Materials 2010;3(10):4695.

19. Dorozhkin SV. Calcium orthophosphate cements for biomedical application. J Mater Sci 2008;43(9): 3028–57.

20. Colon DA, Yoon BV, Russell TA, et al. Assessment of the injection behavior of commercially available bone BSMs for subchondroplasty (R) procedures. Knee 2015;22(6):597–603.

21. Russell TA, Browne TD, Jacofsky M, et al. The problem of fracture fixation augmentation and description of a novel technique and implant for femoral neck stabilization. Tech Orthop 2015;30(1):22–7.

22. Chen WC, Lin JH, Ju CP. Transmission electron microscopic study on setting mechanism of tetracalcium phosphate/dicalcium phosphate anhydrous-based calcium phosphate cement. J Biomed Mater Res A 2003;64(4):664–71.

23. Ginebra MP, Canal C, Espanol M, et al. Calcium phosphate cements as drug delivery materials. Adv Drug Deliv Rev 2012;64(12):1090–110.

24. Albee FH. Studies in bone growth: triple calcium phosphate as a stimulus to osteogenesis. Ann Surg 1920;71(1):32–9.

25. Chow LC. Next generation calcium phosphate-based biomaterials. Dent Mater J 2009;28(1):1–10.

26. Ray RD, Ward AA Jr. A preliminary report on studies of basic calcium phosphate in bone replacement. Surg Forum 1951;429–34.

27. Lange TA, Zerwekh JE, Peek RD, et al. Granular tricalcium phosphate in large cancellous defects. Ann Clin Lab Sci 1986;16(6):467–72.

28. Le Huec JC, Lesprit E, Delavigne C, et al. Tri-calcium phosphate ceramics and allografts as bone substitutes for spinal fusion in idiopathic scoliosis as bone substitutes for spinal fusion in idiopathic scoliosis: comparative clinical results at four years. Acta Orthop Belg 1997;63(3):202–11.

29. Brown WE, Chow LC. A new calcium phosphate water-setting cement. In: Brown, editor. Cements research progress. Westville (OH): American Ceramic Society; 1986. p. 351–79.

30. Brown WE, Chow LC. A new calcium phosphate setting cement. J Dent Res 1983;62:672.

31. Egol KA, Sugi MT, Ong CC, et al. Fracture site augmentation with calcium phosphate cement reduces screw penetration after open reduction-internal fixation of proximal humeral fractures. J Shoulder Elbow Surg 2012;21(6):741–8.

32. Giannoudis PV, Kanakaris NK, Delli Sante E, et al. Acetabular fractures with marginal impaction: mid-term results. Bone Joint J 2013;95B(2):230–8.

33. Johal HS, Buckley RE, Le IL, et al. A prospective randomized controlled trial of a bioresorbable calcium phosphate paste (alpha-BSM) in treatment of displaced intra-articular calcaneal fractures. J Trauma 2009;67(4):875–82.

34. Russell TA, Leighton RK. Comparison of autogenous bone graft and endothermic calcium phosphate cement for defect augmentation in tibial plateau fractures. A multicenter, prospective, randomized study. J Bone Joint Surg Am 2008; 90(10):2057–61.

35. Larsson S, Berg P, Sagerfors M. Augmentation of tibial plateau fractures with calcium phosphate cement: a randomized study using radiostereometry. In Proceedings of the OTA Meeting. Hollywood (FL), 2004.

36. Heinemann S, Rössler S, Lemm M, et al. Properties of injectable ready-to-use calcium phosphate cement based on water-immiscible liquid. Acta Biomater 2013;9(4):6199–207.

37. Ginebra MP, Fernández E, Driessens FCM, et al. Modeling of the hydrolysis of α-tricalcium phosphate. J Am Ceram Soc 1999;82(10):2808–12.

38. McDonald E, Chu T, Tufaga M, et al. Tibial plateau fracture repairs augmented with calcium phosphate cement have higher in situ fatigue strength than those with autograft. J Orthop Trauma 2011;25(2):90–5.

Bone Morphogenetic Protein

Is There Still a Role in Orthopedic Trauma in 2017?

Eric A. Barcak, DO*, Michael J. Beebe, MD

KEYWORDS

- Bone morphogenetic protein • Fracture • Trauma • Nonunion • Complications

---

KEY POINTS

- Recombinant bone morphogenetic protein-2 can be beneficial when treating open tibia fractures, specifically, Gustilo-Anderson type 3 injuries.
- Recombinant bone morphogenetic protein-7 can be beneficial when treating tibia shaft nonunions.
- Off-label use of bone morphogenetic protein is common despite limited evidence to support its use in these settings.
- Increasing reports of bone morphogenetic protein–related complications with off-label use are being described in the orthopedic trauma literature.
- The economic impact of BMP use in fracture care in the United States is unknown.

INTRODUCTION

The discovery of bone morphogenetic proteins (BMP) by Urist[1] in 1965 was met with great optimism. The finding of an osteoinductive compound created the potential for manufacturing a growth factor that would assist with bone formation and healing. Over the years, numerous studies (both animal and human) showed the efficacy of BMP in enhancing bone growth.[2–5] Moreover, many of these studies have found ancillary benefits of BMP, such as decreasing infection rates and time to wound healing.[4] In 2001, the US Food and Drug Administration (FDA) gave marketing clearance for rhBMP-7 (OP-1; Stryker [Stryker Corporation, Kalamazoo, Michigan]) to be used for recalcitrant long bone nonunions. Subsequently, in 2004, rhBMP-2 (INFUSE; Medtronic [Medtronic, Fridley, Minnesota]) was approved for treatment of open tibia shaft fractures. Unfortunately, recent reports of complications have overshadowed these early promising results. Increased wound drainage, excessive bone growth, neuropathy, and even carcinogenesis have been presented as complications after use of BMP.[6–8] Additionally, concern over lack of mechanical strength and the high cost associated with BMP have been cited as shortcomings.[9] Many of the reports on complications occurred after use around the spine; however, there are also reports of complications associated with fracture care.[6,7,10]

Approximately 10 years ago BMP was seen as a miraculous adjuvant to assist with bone growth. However, in the face of an increasing number of complications and a lack of understanding its long-term effects, it is unclear what role BMP has in the current treatment of orthopedic trauma patients. This article to reviews the current recommendations, trends, and associated complications of BMP use in fracture care.

Department of Orthopedic Surgery, University of Tennessee-Campbell Clinic, 1211 Union Avenue #500, Memphis, TN 38104, USA
* Corresponding author.
E-mail address: ebarcak@campbellclinic.com

Orthop Clin N Am 48 (2017) 301–309
http://dx.doi.org/10.1016/j.ocl.2017.03.004
0030-5898/17/© 2017 Elsevier Inc. All rights reserved.

HISTORY AND MECHANISM OF BONE MORPHOGENETIC PROTEIN

BMPs are a part of the transforming growth factor-β superfamily that is responsible for tissue repair and embryogenesis.[11,12] Twenty different BMPs have been discovered with many of them appearing to function in different ways. When acting together, these growth factors are able to provide a signal that causes mesenchymal stem cells to differentiate into osteoblasts, also known as *osteoinduction*. Specific proteins (BMP-2, -6, and -9) work early in the differentiation process, whereas most of the others, including BMP-7, help stimulate the final transition of preosteoblast to osteoblasts.[11]

Urist[1] is credited as being the founder of these growth factors after he implanted decalcified bone within rodent muscle and noticed subsequent bone growth. He defined this phenomenon as *osteoinduction*. In 1988, Johnson and colleagues[13] reported the first clinical outcomes of purified human BMP used to treat femoral nonunions. Eleven of the 12 femoral nonunions treated healed at an average of 4.7 months. Johnson performed additional clinical trials that continued to show promising results.[14,15] However, it became apparent early on that isolating large quantities of BMP from cadaveric bone was difficult and not a viable source for mass scale production.[12] Moreover, the specific dose of BMP required for efficacy was unknown, which led to use of recombinant gene technology to create specific BMPs that show evidence of osteoinduction alone.[12] Both rhBMP-2 (INFUSE) and rhBMP-7 (OP-1) are proteins that are now manufactured in mass quantities via recombinant technology. These proteins are currently the most widely used and most studied of the BMP family. Further studies followed that found that low doses of BMP resulted in minimal bone formation; however, higher doses of BMP can result in excessive bone formation and even bone resorption secondary to osteoclast activation.[11] Termaat and colleagues[11] explained that "The dose of BMP needed for clinical efficacy must overcome a threshold, and the dose-response curve becomes steeper as one progresses from rodent to nonhuman primate." The specific reason for this is still unclear. At this time, the current recommended doses of BMP-2 and BMP-7 are more than 1000 times greater than those of native concentrations.

TREATMENT OF ACUTE FRACTURES

The treatment of open fractures is associated with high complications rates and poor functional outcomes. Loss of soft tissue and bone in these injuries may lead to delayed healing and nonunion. Much of the clinical research with BMP use in acute extremity injuries involves open fractures, specifically, open tibia fractures.

In 2002, the BMP-2 Evaluation in Surgery for Tibial Trauma (BESTT) trial was performed to determine the safety and efficacy of rhBMP-2 in the treatment of open tibia shaft fractures fixed with both reamed and unreamed intramedullary nails (IMN).[4] Four hundred fifty patients with open tibia shaft fractures were randomly divided into 3 groups:

1. The standard of care group (IMN plus soft tissue management)
2. The standard of care with 0.75 mg/mL of rhBMP-2
3. The standard of care with 1.50 mg/mL of rhBMP-2

The authors found that the group with 1.50 mg/mL of rhBMP-2 had significantly fewer reoperations, infections, wound complications, and hardware failures. Additionally, the group with the 1.50 mg/mL dose had faster healing times. At 1 year follow-up, the adverse events in the BMP group were similar to what was seen in a normal trauma setting. The authors stated that rhBMP-2 is a "novel adjunct" and advantageous when compared with the standard of care when treating long bone fractures. However, other investigators noted the disproportionate amount of patients in the control group that received unreamed IMN when compared with the study group.[16] The effect of reaming when treating tibia fractures with IMN has been well studied. The Study to Prospectively Evaluate Reamed Intramedullary Nails in Patients with Tibial Fractures (SPRINT) trial[17] found that the reaming is a strong confounding variable to consider in the BESTT trial results.

In 2006, Swiontkowski and colleagues[18] combined the data from the BESST trial with data from another prospective, randomized trial using the same methods. Patients from 2 subgroups were analyzed:

1. 131 patients with Gustilo-Anderson type 3A or 3B fractures
2. 113 patients treated with reamed IMN

This analysis found significant improvements in secondary procedures and infections in those from the first subgroup receiving rhBMP-2 at a concentration of 1.50 mg/mL. The second subgroup showed no difference between those that received rhBMP-2 and those that did not, but a trend toward improved outcomes in the treatment group was noted by the authors (P>.30). The study concluded that rhBMP-2 significantly reduces the frequency of bone grafting and secondary procedures when treating Gustilo-Anderson type 3 open tibia fractures. However, the authors admit that the study was not originally designed for a subgroup analysis and that the data alone "should be viewed with caution."

McKee and colleagues[19] evaluated the role of rhBMP-7 (OP1) in the treatment of open tibia fractures treated with IMN. One hundred twenty-four patients were randomly assigned to a control group (simple closure) and compared with those who had simple closure with the addition of 3.4 mg of rhBMP-7 at the fracture site. Patients in the rhBMP-7 group showed significant improvements in rates of reoperation, overall pain, and functional scores. No adverse events were associated with rhBMP-7 use. These data was presented at the Orthopaedic Trauma Association's annual meeting in 2013 but have not been published to date.

Most recently, Aro and colleagues[16] performed a randomized trial of 277 patients to evaluate the role of rhBMP-2 in the treatment of open tibia shaft fractures fixed with only reamed IMN. In contrast to the BESST study, no significant difference was found between the groups. A notable difference between the 2 studies was the higher proportion of Gustilo-Anderson type 3 injuries in the BESTT study (43% vs 32%). Additionally, the BESST study had a lower percentage (22%) of Gustilo-Anderson type 1 injuries than the study by Aro and colleagues (29%). This discrepancy could explain the different outcomes presented, as Gustilo-Anderson type 3 injuries have been associated with higher reoperation rates.[20] A trend toward increased deep infection rates was seen in the rhBMP-2 group in the study by Aro and colleagues, but this did not reach significance (P = .0645). This finding differs from those of other studies that suggest that BMP may assist with decreasing deep infection rates. The reason for this finding remains unclear. The authors suggest that it may be associated with the surgical technique, as many of the infections in the treatment group occurred in Gustilo-Anderson type 1 injuries. The collagen delivery device for the BMP could have potentially placed pressure on these small wounds leading to necrosis and possible infection. Notably, the authors state that although the treatment had a higher number of infections, the overall fracture healing rate was not affected.

A recent meta-analysis of randomized trials was published discussing BMP use in open tibia fractures. Four studies that specifically analyzed BMP use in open tibia fractures were evaluated.[21] The authors concluded that there is some evidence for improved union rates in patients treated with BMP versus standard of care; however, "no clear answers" were established in the study. Final recommendations included the need for well-designed randomized, controlled trials. Box 1 summarizes the data for BMP use in open tibia fractures.

In addition to open tibia fractures, some investigators also evaluated the effects of BMP on acute closed tibial shaft fractures. A double-blinded, randomized, controlled trial of 369 patients with closed tibia shaft fractures was performed.[22] Patients were randomly assigned to the standard of care (reamed, locked IMN), the standard of care plus 1 mg/mL of rhBMP-2 in an injectable calcium phosphate matrix (CPM), the standard of care plus 2 mg/mL of rhBMP-2 with CPM, and the standard of care with CPM only. The main outcome measures were time to union and time to return of normal function. The study was terminated early after 180 patients underwent interim analysis at 6 months. No difference in healing was seen between the groups in terms of healing or return to function; however, a significantly higher number of severe complications, edema, and deep venous thrombosis was seen in the treatment groups when compared with the standard of care. Of note, the rates of infection and compartment syndrome were comparable among the groups and with previously published data.

The authors concluded that time to union and return to function were not significantly reduced by adding BMP-2/CPM when treating patients with closed tibial shaft fractures with reamed IMN. The possibility of an injectable adjuvant

---

Box 1
Bone morphogenetic protein use in open tibia fractures

1. rhBMP-2 may assist with healing of open tibia fractures.

2. Evidence suggests that rhBMP-2 is more effective in severe open wounds (Gustilo-Anderson type III) than in less severe open wounds (Gustilo-Anderson type I).

3. There is conflicting evidence that BMP improves infection rates.

4. There is a need for well-designed, better-controlled, randomized trials.

that can assist with fracture healing is a desirable concept. Unfortunately, at this time, there is limited clinical evidence to suggest benefit in its current form.

NONUNION

Autologous bone grafting has traditionally been used to assist with healing when treating nonunions because it provides not only structural support but also osteoinductive and osteogenic factors to assist with healing. Additional benefits include limited immunogenicity and possibly decreased monetary cost, albeit with the expense of possible donor site morbidity.[23] Although autograft has shown benefits in the treatment of bony deficits, it has come under scrutiny for increasing the risk of complications and donor site pain.[24] Consequently, the idea of an implantable osteoinductive growth factor that can avoid donor site morbidity while acting as an adjuvant to osteoconductive fillers has become increasingly popular. This has led to numerous studies looking at BMP and its efficacy when treating nonunions and fractures with bone loss.

Fracture nonunion is often a multifactorial problem that can be difficult to treat. The etiology of many nonunions, particularly oligotrophic or atrophic variants, can be the result of a compromised healing response that prevents bony union. Additionally, many nonunions can result from significant bone loss at the time of injury. BMPs have been studied in each of these scenarios.

Friedlaender and colleagues[5] studied the efficacy of rhBMP-7 (OP1) in the treatment of tibial nonunions. One hundred twenty-two patients with tibia nonunions were treated with reamed IMN and randomly assigned to autograft versus OP1 implantation at the nonunion site. Similar rates of healing were seen between the 2 groups. Additionally, a trend toward lower infection rates was seen in the rhBMP-7 group. Twenty percent of the autograft cohort had continued pain at the donor site. The authors concluded that rhBMP-7 is a safe and reasonable alternative to autologous bone grafting when treating tibial nonunions without the risk of donor site pain.

An additional multicenter study by Kanakaris and colleagues[25] evaluated 68 patients with aseptic tibial nonunions treated with 3.5 mg of rhBMP-7 mixed with 1 g of collagen carrier. Surgeons were permitted to use autograft (36%) if deemed necessary to assist as a "graft expander." They achieved a 90% union rate and

had no complications or adverse events associated with BMP application.

Similar studies continue to show promising results with long bone nonunions.[26] Unfortunately, when comparing these studies, there is variability in study design and inclusion criteria. Additionally, the types of nonunions treated, along with the specific definitions for nonunion, is inconsistent, making these studies difficult to compare.

A meta-analysis presented in 2014 stated that overall union rates were similar between BMP-treated and non–BMP-treated patients with nonunions.[27] However, when looking specifically at rhBMP-7 use in tibial nonunions, the only FDA-approved indication, there was a significantly higher union rate in the BMP group. Additionally, a decrease in secondary interventions was seen in nonunions treated with BMP when compared with control. However, the analysis showed higher levels of significance in lower-level studies when compared with level 1 studies. This finding likely indicates confounding factors introduced during the lower-level studies, further blurring the findings.

OFF-LABEL USE OF BONE MORPHOGENETIC PROTEIN IN NONUNION TREATMENT

Although most of the currently published research of BMP use in nonunions looks specifically at tibia fractures, there is a growing trend of off-label use for nonunions in other areas of the body. A recent prospective, randomized cohort study evaluated 49 patients with aseptic radial or ulnar diaphyseal nonunions.[28] Each patient was treated with compression plating and autologous bone grafting. In addition, 24 of the patients had either rhBMP-2 or rhBMP-7 added to their treatment at the time of surgery. No significant differences in healing or complications were seen between the 2 groups. Additionally, clinical outcome measures were similar in each cohort.

Another recent retrospective cohort study evaluated long bone nonunions in the upper extremity.[29] All fractures were treated with compression plating along with application of rhBMP-7 at the time of surgery. Cortical strut grafts were used based on surgeon discretion to assist with fixation; however, no other osteobiologics were used at the fracture site. Eighty-nine percent of the patients went on to union by 1 year. Reported complications include 1 deep infection, 4 superficial infections, a radial nerve palsy, a cervical radiculopathy, and a case of diffuse hand paresthesias. The only complication that required an additional surgery was the deep infection. No specific adverse events occurred as a result of BMP application.

These studies provide promising results, but similar to previous BMP-related nonunion studies, they are difficult to compare.

BONE MORPHOGENETIC PROTEIN-7 VERSUS BONE MORPHOGENETIC PROTEIN-2 IN THE TREATMENT OF NONUNIONS

A recent single-center study compared BMP-7 and BMP-2 in the treatment of long bone nonunions of the upper and lower extremities.[30] The BMP-2 group showed improved radiographic healing (*P*<.001), time to healing (*P*<.001), and time to weight bearing (*P*<.001). Of note, the BMP-7 cohort had an older patient population, and more patients that had previously been treated for infections. The authors admit that this could be a cofounding variable in their results. Additionally, many of these nonunions were treated with different types of surgical fixation and involved diverse areas of the body. Interestingly, a comparison of healing times of patients with previous infections also showed the BMP-2 cohort had significant improvements in healing when compared with the BMP-7 cohort. Although the study provides promising results, BMP-2 use in nonunion care remains off label. **Box 2** summarizes BMP use in the treatment of nonunions.

COMPLICATIONS

Although the initial results of BMP use were promising, more recent studies are reporting complications with their use. In a 2011 Orthopaedic Research Society Forum, the specific role of rhBMP-2 in orthopedics was discussed. Specific concerns over the massive doses of rhBMP-2, when compared with the physiologic dose, along with underreporting of complications, were major concerns. It was argued that the results of many of the BMP studies, specifically in the spine literature, may be "too good to be true."[31] Overall, many of the previously discussed articles do not include BMP-related complications associated with fracture care. Nonunions and open fractures are difficult problems to treat and are classically fraught with complications. Understandably, it is difficult to specifically associate BMP use with adverse events in this patient population, especially in small series. There are a few studies and case reports published that discuss specific complications associated with BMP use and fracture care.

WOUND DRAINAGE

In 2014, Chan and colleagues[10] presented 2 cohorts of patients who underwent reconstruction procedures or who had acute open fractures. The 2 cohorts were similar except that one of the groups was treated with rhBMP-2 during the time of surgery. An overall increased rate of wound drainage was found in the rhBMP-2 group. Interestingly, most of these patients (72%) were successfully treated conservatively without additional intervention. Moreover, the rhBMP-2 cohort showed improved rates in healing and postoperative infection, despite the increased wound drainage. These findings are similar to the findings presented in the BESTT trial.

A case report was also published of 2 patients who were treated for long bone nonunions with fixation and rhBMP-2.[32] Both patients had acute postoperative swelling that was clinically suspicious for infection and resulted in further operations. Cultures were negative in both patients. Intraoperative evaluation found severe tissue inflammation near the BMP sponge.

Ritting and colleagues[7] presented a similar case report of "massive inflammatory reaction" in a pediatric patient treated with BMP-2 and fixation for a symptomatic ulnar nonunion.

If these studies are showing related complications, then there seems to be a spectrum of tissue reaction that can occur with BMP use. Similar reports of wound drainage and inflammation have also been presented in the spine literature.[33] The specific reason for the reaction is unknown; however, an immune-modulated inflammatory response is one of the proposed mechanisms.[10] The specific clinical relevance of this phenomenon remains undetermined at this time, but surgeons should be aware of the reaction and the likeness to postsurgical infection on examination.

Box 2
Bone morphogenetic protein use in the treatment of nonunions

1. rhBMP-7 can be useful when treating tibial shaft nonunions.

2. Off-label use of rhBMP-2 and rhBMP-7 is common, although there is limited evidence to suggest its efficacy in these settings.

3. There is variability in study design and definitions in many of the BMP-related nonunion studies.

4. There is a need for well-designed clinical trials of BMP use in the treatment of nonunions.

NEUROPATHY

Neuropathy is a commonly reported complication of BMP use in the spine.[34] Interestingly, a recent case report was published in the *Journal of Bone and Joint Surgery*.[35] A patient was treated with open reduction and internal fixation along with rhBMP-2 for a nonunion of a clavicle fracture. The patient subsequently had a motor and sensory brachial plexus palsy postoperatively. No evidence of mass effect was seen on postfixation imaging to suggest compression. The authors attributed the nerve injury to BMP use, although the specific mechanism of injury is unclear. Ultimately, the patient's nerve injury healed, without intervention, 2 years after surgery. Previous animal studies have associated "axonal drop out" with BMP use near peripheral nerves; however, the most recent case report is the only clinical evidence we could find of this complication in fracture care.[36]

ECTOPIC BONE

Increasing reports of excess bone growth have been associated with BMP application. A comparison of 2 cohorts of patients with tibial plateau fractures treated with either open reduction internal fixation (ORIF; 23 patients) or ORIF plus rhBMP-2 (17 patients) were evaluated at a minimum of 12 months.[6] The risk of symptomatic heterotopic ossification development was significantly higher in the rhBMP-2 group when compared with control (P<.001). Forty percent of these patients had clinically significant bone formation that required additional surgery. Of note, no difference in maintenance of reduction was seen between the 2 cohorts.

Another study followed up with 6 patients who underwent surgery for failed ORIF of scaphoid fractures.[37] All patients were treated with repeat ORIF, rhBMP-2, and autograft. Four of the 6 patients showed radiographic evidence of heterotopic ossification. One of these patients required surgery to remove excess bone secondary to loss of motion.

Many of the higher-powered studies involving BMP were performed on diaphyseal fractures of long bones, particularly in the lower extremity. Symptomatic heterotopic bone usually occurs when it's adjacent to a joint and therefore may not have been reported. Careful consideration of BMP use near articulations should be taken until further studies can be completed.

CARCINOGENESIS

Transforming growth factor-β family proteins are known to play a role in tumor progression and suppression. Subsequently, there is concern that BMP administered at superphysiologic doses could result in carcinogenesis.

A previous randomized investigational device exemption study that included patients (N = 518) undergoing spinal fusion for lumbar degenerative disease was conducted to evaluate rhBMP-2 in lumbar fusions.[38] One group received Medtronic's Amplify product, a combination of rhBMP-2 (40 mg) with a proprietary compression resistant matrix, whereas the other group received iliac crest bone graft. The primary outcome measure of the study was to evaluate serious complications related to the product. No patients had a history of cancer before surgery. At 2-year follow up, 8 patients were found to have cancer in the Amplify group versus 2 in the control group (P<.0026). Five years later, the FDA reported a total of 13 cancers in the study group versus 4 in the control group. None of these new cancers were considered related to the study procedure.[39] Carragee and colleagues[8] provided an excellent analysis of the data at both 2 and 5 years. Ultimately, they concluded that a high dose of rhBMP-2 (40 mg) in lumbar spine fusions was associated with the risk of new cancer, and the product was thus rejected by the FDA.

After this evidence was revealed, a retrospective study of 146,278 patients who underwent lumbar spinal fusion was performed.[40] Roughly 22,000 of these patients received rhBMP during their procedures. In contrast to the Amplify study, at an average follow-up of 4.7 years, 15.4% of the BMP cohort and 17% of the control, had a new cancer (hazard ratio, 0.98; 95% confidence interval, 0.95 to 1.02). The authors concluded from their analysis that there was no evidence that administration of rhBMP during lumbar fusion increases cancer risk.

Multiple systematic reviews have also been written over the last few years discussing BMP and cancer risk. Devine and colleagues[41] evaluated 5 peer-reviewed studies and 2 FDA safety summaries of carcinogenesis associated with rhBMP-2 and rhBMP-7 use. They concluded that cancer risk may be associated with increasing doses of rhBMP-2; however, there is still a need for longer follow-up in many of the patients. In a similar study, Skovrilj and colleagues[42] performed a systematic review of 99 studies (both human and animal) that directly looked at rhBMP-2 and cancer. No studies found that BMP caused cancer de novo. However, 43 studies suggested that BMP enhanced tumor function. Eighteen of the studies also suggested BMP suppressed malignancy, further clouding the picture.

Unfortunately, there are no studies documenting cancer risk in patients treated with BMP for fracture care. Although the potential benefits of BMP are evident, it is imperative that health care providers discuss the potential complications associated with their use with their patients.

IMMUNOGENICITY

At this time, many of the collagen carriers of BMP are immunogenic.[11] The creation of specific antibodies against BMP may be problematic in certain patients, especially if BMP is used in more than one setting. Additionally, as previously discussed, these antibodies may play a role in the acute swelling and wound drainage seen in some patients treated with BMP.[10] The presence of antibodies has been positively correlated with high doses of BMP, but this presence is not apparent in all patients.[5] Multiple spine studies evaluated the immunogenicity of BMP and its relation to bone healing and complications.[43,44] Although these reactions do occur in certain patients, they seem to be transient and not directly correlated with clinical outcomes. Unfortunately, it is still unclear why this reaction occurs in certain patients. Moreover, complications of BMP use in more than one setting remains unknown.

COST ANALYSIS/ECONOMICS

More than ever before, the cost of specific treatments is being scrutinized in our health care system. The specific cost of BMP is volume dependent with large volumes priced up to $5,000.[45] However, extended work absence combined with additional medical costs associated with repeat surgery should also be considered. Dahabreh and Giannoudis[46] performed a study comparing the cost implications of tibia nonunions treated with autologous bone grafting versus BMP-7. The total costs of surgical treatment, hospital stay, and follow-up were analyzed. The average cost of tibia nonunions treated with autologous bone grafting was 6.7% higher than those treated with BMP-7. This finding did not reach statistical significance. In another study, Garrison and colleagues[47] stated that the "the cost-effectiveness of additional BMP may be improved if the price of BMP is reduced or if BMP is used in severe cases." Final recommendations include the need for further trials with economic evaluation. As Argintar and colleagues[45] noted in their review, many of the cost analysis studies were performed in Europe. The specific economic impact has not been determined in a United States cohort.

SUMMARY

Recombinant BMP is an innovative tool to assist with bone healing. Some studies found improvements in healing and infection rates among patients with acute fractures and nonunions. However, BMP is certainly not a panacea and is not without risk of complications. Moreover, the specific economic impact of BMP in the United States and long-term effects of the protein are still unknown. There is a need for well-designed clinical trials to further investigate their use. Health care providers should discuss both the potential benefits and pitfalls of using this adjuvant therapy with their patients before use.

REFERENCES

1. Urist MR. Bone: formation by autoinduction. Science 1965;150:893–9.
2. Den Boer FC, Bramer JA, Blokhuis TJ, et al. Effect of recombinant human osteogenic protein-1 on the healing of a freshly closed diaphyseal fracture. Bone 2002;31:158–64.
3. Mizumoto Y, Moseley T, Drews M, et al. Acceleration of regenerate ossification during distraction osteogenesis with recombinant human bone morphogenetic protein-7. J Bone Joint Surg Am 2003;85(Suppl 3):124–30.
4. Govender S, Csimma C, Genant HK, et al, BMP-2 Evaluation in Surgery for Tibial Trauma (BESTT) Study Group. Recombinant human bone morphogenetic protein-2 for treatment of open tibial fractures: a prospective, controlled, randomized study of four hundred and fifty patients. J Bone Joint Surg Am 2002;84:2123–34.
5. Friedlaender GE, Perry CR, Cole JD, et al. Osteogenic protein-1 (bone morphogenetic protein-(7) in the treatment of tibial nonunions. J Bone Joint Surg Am 2001;83-A(Suppl 1(Pt 2)):S151–8.
6. Sreevathsa B, Omesh P, Hawkes D, et al. Complications of recombinant human BMP-2 for treating complex tibial plateau fractures: a preliminary report. Clin Orthop Relat Res 2009;467(12):3257–62.
7. Ritting A, Weber E, Lee M. Exaggerated inflammatory response and bony resorption from BMP-2 use in a pediatric forearm nonunion. J Hand Surg 2012;37(2):316–21.
8. Carragee E, Chu G, Rohatgi R, et al. Cancer risk after use of recombinant bone morphogenetic protein-2 for spinal arthrodesis. J Bone Joint Surg Am 2013;95(17):1537–45.

9. Axelrad T, Kakar S, Einhorn T. Biological and biophysical technologies for the enhancement of fracture repair. In: Bucholz R, Court-Brown C, Heckman J, et al, editors. Rockwood and green's fractures in the adult, V1. 7th edition. Philadelphia: Lippincott Williams and Wilkins; 2010. p. 11–113.

10. Chan D, Garland J, Infante A, et al. Wound complications associated with bone morphogenetic protein-2 in orthopaedic trauma surgery. J Orthop Trauma 2014;28(10):599–604.

11. Termaat MF, Boer D, Bakker FC, et al. Current concepts review, bone morphogenic proteins, development and clinical efficacy in the treatment of fractures and bone defects. J Bone Joint Surg 2005;87-A(6):1367–78.

12. De Long W, Einhorn T, Koval K, et al. Current concepts review, bone grafts an bone graft substitutes in orthopaedic trauma surgery. A critical analysis. J Bone Joint Surg 2007;89-A(3):649–58.

13. Johnson EE, Urist MR, Finerman GA. Distal metaphyseal tibial nonunion. Deformity and bone loss treated by open reduction, internal fixation, and human bone morphogenetic protein (hBMP). Clin Orthop Relat Res 1990;250:234–40.

14. Johnson EE, Urist MR, Finerman GA. Repair of segmental defects of the tibia with cancellous bone grafts augmented with human bone morphogenetic protein. A preliminary report. Clin Orthop Relat Res 1988;236:249–57.

15. Johnson EE, Urist MR, Finerman GA. Bone morphogenetic protein augmentation grafting of resistant femoral nonunions. A preliminary report. Clin Orthop Relat Res 1988;230:257–65.

16. Aro H, Govender S, Patel A, et al. Recombinant human bone morphogenetic protein-2: a randomized trial in open tibial fractures treated with reamed nail fixation. J Bone Joint Surg Am 2011;93:801–8.

17. Bhandari M, Guyatt G, Tornetta, et al. Randomized trial of reamed and unreamed intramedullary nailing of tibial shaft fractures. J Bone Joint Surg Am 2008;90:2567–78.

18. Swiontkowski M, Aro H, Donell S, et al. Recombinant human bone morphogenetic protein-2 in open tibial fractures. a subgroup analysis of data combined from two prospective randomized studies. J Bone Joint Surg Am 2006;88A(6):1258–65.

19. McKee MD, Schemitsch EH, Waddell JP, et al. The effect of human recombinant bone morphogenic protein (rhBMP-7) on the healing of open tibial shaft fractures: results of a multi-center, prospective, randomized clinical trial. Read at the Annual Meeting of the American Academy of Orthopaedic Surgeons; 2003; New Orleans, LA, February 5–8, 2003.

20. Harris I, Lyons M. Reoperation rate in diaphyseal tibia fractures. ANZ J Surg 2005;75:1041–4.

21. Dai J, Li L, Jiang C, et al. Bone morphogenetic protein for the healing of tibial fracture: a meta-analysis of randomized controlled trials. PLoS One 2015;10(10):e0141670.

22. Lyon T, Scheele W, Bhandari M, et al. Efficacy and safety of recombinant human bone morphogenetic protein-2/calcium phosphate matrix for closed tibial diaphyseal fracture a double-blind, randomized, controlled phase-II/III trial. J Bone Joint Surg Am 2013;95:2088–96.

23. Blokhuis T, Calori G, Schmidmaier G. Autograft versus BMPs for the treatment of non-unions: what is the evidence? Injury 2013;44:S40–2.

24. Arrington ED, Smith WJ, Chambers HG, et al. Complications of iliac crest bone graft harvesting. Clin Orthop Relat Res 1996;329:300–9.

25. Kanakaris N, Calori G, Verdonk R, et al. Application of BMP-7 to tibial non-unions: a 3-year multicenter experience. Injury 2008;39(2):S83–90.

26. Zimmermann G, Moghaddam A, Wagner C, et al. Clinical experience with bone morphogenetic protein 7 (BMP 7) in nonunions of long bones. Unfallchirurg 2006;109(7):528–37 [in German].

27. Schenker M, Yannascoli S, Donegan D, et al. Bone morphogenetic protein and fractures: a meta-analysis. ORS 2014 Annual Meeting Poster No: 0638, New Orleans, LA, March 15-18, 2014.

28. von Rüden C, Morgenstern M, Hierholzer C, et al. The missing effect of human recombinant bone morphogenetic proteins BMP-2 and BMP-7 in surgical treatment of aseptic forearm nonunion. Injury 2016;47:919–24.

29. Morison M, Vicente M, Schemitsch E, et al. The treatment of atrophic, recalcitrant long-bone nonunion in the upper extremity with human recombinant bone morphogenetic protein-7 (rhBMP-7) and plate fixation: a retrospective review. Injury 2016;47(2):356–63.

30. Conway J, Shabtai L, Bauernschub A, et al. BMP-7 Versus BMP-2 for the treatment of long bone nonunion. Orthopedics 2014;37(12):31049–57.

31. Stanton T. Lesson learned: what the BMP trials controversy has taught us. Available at: http://www.aaos.org/News/The_Daily_Edition_of_AAOS_Now/2012/Thursday,_February_9/AAOS9_2_9/?ssopc=1. Accessed February 10, 2016.

32. Young A, Mirarchi A. Soft tissue swelling associated with the use of RhBMP2 in long bone nonunions. J Orthop Case Rep 2015;5(3):18–21.

33. Saulle D, Fu KM, Smith JS. Multiple-day drainage when using bone morphogenic protein for long-segment thoracolumbar fusions is associated with low rates of wound complications. World Neurosurg 2013;80(1–2):204–7.

34. Chrastil J, Low J, Whang P, et al. Complications associated with the use of the recombinant human bone morphogenetic proteins for posterior

interbody fusions of the lumbar spine. Spine 2013;
38(16):E1020–7.

35. Matthews J, Margolis D, Wu E, et al. Brachial plexopathy following use of recombinant human BMP-2 for treatment of atrophic delayed union of the clavicle. JBJS Case Connect 2015;5(3):e81.

36. Margolis DS, We EW, Truchan LM. Axonal loss in murine peripheral nerves following exposure to recombinant human bone morphogenetic protein-2 in an absorbable collagen sponge. J Bone Joint Surg Am 2014;95(7):611–9.

37. Brannan P, Gaston G, Loeffler B, et al. Complications with the use of BMP-2 in scaphoid nonunion surgery. J Hand Surg 2016;41(5):602–8.

38. United States of America Department of Health and Human Services Food and Drug Administration. Food and Drug Administration executive summary for P050036Medtronic's AmplifyTM rhBMP-2 matrix orthopaedic and rehabilitation devices advisory panel. Available at: http://www.fda.gov.ezproxy.uthsc.edu/downloads/Advisory Committees/CommitteesMeetingMater. Accessed February 10, 2016.

39. Orthopaedic and Rehabilitation Devices Panel, Medical Devices Advisory Committee, Center for Devices and Radiological Health, U.S. Food and Drug Administration. Available at: http://www.fda.gov.ezproxy.uthsc.edu/downloads/Advisory Committees/CommitteesMeetingMaterials/Medical DevicesAdvisoryCommittee/OrthopaedicandRehabi. Accessed February 10, 2016.

40. Cooper G, Kou T. Risk of cancer after lumbar fusion surgery with recombinant human bone morphogenic protein-2 (rh-BMP-2). Spine 2013;38(21):1862–8.

41. Devine JG, Dettori JR, France JC, et al. The use of rhBMP in spine surgery: is there a cancer risk? Evid Based Spine Care J 2012;3(2):35–41.

42. Skovrilj B, Koehler SM, Anderson PA, et al. Association between BMP-2 and carcinogenicity. Spine (Phila Pa 1976) 2015;40(23):1862–71.

43. Hwang C, Vaccaro A, Lawrence J, et al. Immunogenecity of bone morphogenetic proteins. J Nuerosurgery Spine 2009;10(5):443–51.

44. Burkus JK, Gornet MF, Glassman SD, et al. Blood serum antibody analysis and long-term follow-up of patients treated with recombinant human bone morphogenetic protein-2 in the lumbar spine. Spine (Phila Pa 1976) 2011;36(25):2158–67.

45. Argintar E, Edwards S, Delahay J. Bone morphogenic proteins in orthopaedic trauma surgery. Injury 2011;42(8):730–4.

46. Dahabreh Z, Giannoudis P. A cost analysis of treatment of tibial fracture non-unions: a comparative studie between autologous iliac crest bone grafting and bone morphogenetic protein-7. Orthopaedic Proceedings, 2012, February 23.

47. Garrison K, Donell S, Ryder J, et al. Clinical effectiveness and cost-effectiveness of bone morphogenetic proteins in the non-healing of fractures and spinal fusion: a systematic review. Health Technol Assess 2007;11(30):1–150, iii–iv.

Role of Bone Marrow Aspirate in Orthopedic Trauma

Patrick C. Schottel, MD[a],*, Stephen J. Warner, MD, PhD[b]

KEYWORDS

- Bone marrow aspirate • Bone marrow aspirate concentrate • BMAC • Nonunion • Hernigou

KEY POINTS

- Bone marrow aspirate contains mesenchymal stem cells (MSCs) capable of promoting the formation of bone.
- Bone marrow is ideally aspirated from the iliac crest using small syringes in multiple small volume aliquots.
- Determining the iliac crest harvest location and whether to concentrate the aspirate is at the surgeon's discretion; a greater number of injected MSCs is associated with better healing.
- Clinical case series have reported that bone marrow aspirate injection has a success of 75% to 90% in treating atrophic tibial nonunions.

INTRODUCTION

The adult skeleton possesses 2 types of bone marrow: yellow and red. Yellow marrow has undergone adipose involution and is inactive. The red marrow possesses hematopoietic cells as well as 2 known populations of adult stem cells.[1] Hematopoietic stem cells give rise to all cell components of circulating blood, such as erythrocytes, lymphocytes, neutrophils, and thrombocytes. The other stem cell population consists of mesenchymal stem cells (MSCs), which are also known as marrow stromal cells. MSCs have the potential to differentiate into connective tissue cells such as osteoblasts, osteocytes, adipocytes, and chondrocytes. The ability of MSCs to differentiate into bone-producing cells has led to interest in their clinical use in orthopedic trauma to improve fracture healing and to treat bone defects. Numerous in vivo animal studies as well clinical human case series have reported the successful use of MSCs or MSC-containing bone marrow aspirate.

This review summarizes the basic science and clinical results of using MSCs and MSC-containing bone marrow aspirate to increase bone formation in the setting of a nonunion or a critical sized defect. It also reviews the technique of aspirating bone marrow and the various ways of increasing the MSC concentration of the aspirate.

BASIC SCIENCE

The critical component of bone marrow aspirate for use in orthopedic trauma is its population of osteoprogenitor cells. MSCs reside in bone marrow and are multipotent cells with the ability to differentiate into osteoprogenitor or chondroprogenitor cells based on molecular signals from their local environment. Osteoprogenitor cells can then differentiate into osteoblasts in

Disclosure Statement: Neither author has any relationship with a commercial company that has a direct financial interest in subject matter or materials discussed in article or with a company making a competing product.
[a] Department of Orthopaedic Surgery and Rehabilitation, University of Vermont College of Medicine, 95 Carrigan Drive, Burlington, VT 05405, USA; [b] Department of Orthopaedic Surgery, University of Texas Health Science Center at Houston, 6400 Fannin Street, Houston, TX 77030, USA
* Corresponding author. 192 Tilley Drive, South Burlington, VT 05403.
E-mail address: Patrick.Schottel@uvmhealth.org

response to surrounding cytokines and growth factors.[2,3] The differentiation of osteoprogenitor cells and their ability to promote bone formation is augmented by the osteoinductive factors also contained within bone marrow aspirate.[4]

Numerous basic science animal studies have investigated the ability of MSCs to stimulate bone formation. A recent systematic review by Gianakos reported the pooled results of 35 animal studies where bone marrow aspirate concentrate (BMAC) was used to treat critical sized bone defects.[5] The reviewed studies used different animal models, including rabbits, rats, mice, goats, canines, sheep, and pigs. They found that, of the studies that reported their results statistically, 100% (14/14) found significantly greater radiographic evidence of osteogenesis, 81% (13/16) showed significantly increased mean bone volume using micro-CT scanning, and 90% (19/21) found significantly more bone formation based on histologic analysis versus control groups. The limitations of these studies are the wide variation in the animal and bone defect models used as well as the unknown translatability of their findings to human clinical scenarios. However, numerous clinical outcome studies have been published and their findings are comparable with these animal model results.

CLINICAL OUTCOMES

The clinical application of bone marrow aspirate in orthopedic trauma is a relatively new development. The majority of the published studies regarding the clinical outcomes of patients treated with bone marrow aspirate are case series treating nonunions, especially of the tibia. However, bone marrow may have a role not only in delayed or nonunited fractures, but also in certain acute fracture cases.

Acute Fractures
To our knowledge, no published studies have reported the use of bone marrow aspirate in the management of acute fractures. However, there is some evidence that bone marrow aspirate combined with allograft or a collagen scaffold may have the same osteogenic capability as autograft,[6,7] and therefore could potentially be substituted in acute fracture cases with an osseous defect where primary bone grafting is indicated. Hernigou and colleagues[6] evaluated 20 patients with acetabular defects secondary to osteolysis after total hip arthroplasty. Revision of the acetabular component included grafting the osteolytic defect with either autograft,

allograft, or allograft with bone marrow aspirate. All patients later underwent a re-revision for femoral component failure after a mean of 10 years from acetabular grafting. At that time, the area of prior acetabular grafting was evaluated to quantify the MSC content of the graft as well as to perform a histologic analysis of the bone. They found that the cohort of allograft with bone marrow aspirate had a significantly higher concentration of MSCs and demonstrated increased new bone formation compared with the other 2 groups. They concluded that allograft combined with bone marrow aspirate is a reasonable alternative to autograft and had similar osteogenic capability.

We currently perform grafting of acute fractures using allograft and bone marrow aspirate for cases with small to medium bone defects either in patients who have evidence of significant metabolic bone disease causing reduced quality of their autograft (eg, renal osteodystrophy, history of prolonged bisphosphonate use) or in patients who cannot undergo an iliac crest bone harvest or reamer irrigator aspirator (DePuy Synthes, West Chester, PA) procedure for various reasons (Fig. 1). The preferred clinical scenarios when to use the technique of using bone marrow aspirate alone or mixed with allograft in acute fracture treatment are continuing to evolve.

Delayed or Nonunited Fractures
Most literature about bone marrow aspirate use in orthopedic trauma has focused on the successful treatment of delayed or nonunited fractures of the upper and lower extremities. However, the personality of the nonunion and host need to be evaluated thoroughly to determine the potential contribution of infection, metabolic abnormalities, mechanical instability, and status of the surrounding soft tissues before choosing the appropriate treatment. Bone marrow aspirate injection has been shown to have a potential role in the treatment of aseptic, atrophic nonunions with acceptable alignment and minimal gap, or displacement between fracture fragments.[1]

Tibial nonunion treatment with bone marrow aspirate has been well-documented and found to be successful in 75% to 90% of reported tibial nonunion case series (Fig. 2).[8–12] Connolly and colleagues[8] published one of the first studies using bone marrow grafting to treat delayed unions and nonunions percutaneously.[13] Their cohort included 20 tibial nonunions that were treated initially with various techniques, including casting, external fixation, and

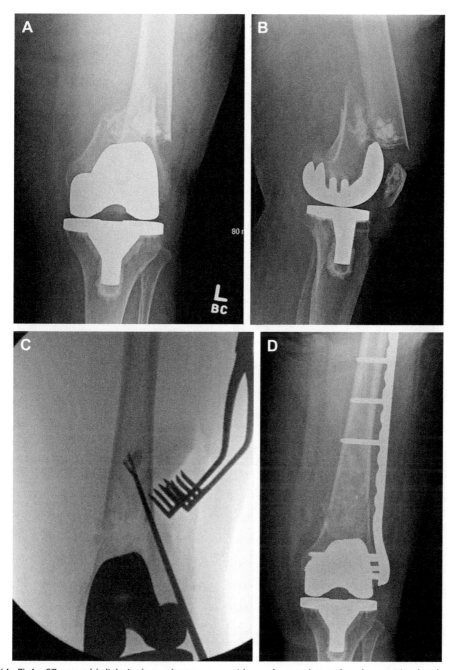

Fig. 1. (A, B) An 87-year-old dialysis-dependent woman with renal osteodystrophy who sustained a closed distal femoral periprosthetic fracture. A biopsy performed at an outside institution of the intramedullary chondroid mass before fracture confirmed it to be a benign enchondroma. (C) An intralesional excision was performed and the defect was filled with bone marrow aspirate combined with allograft. (D) A postoperative anteroposterior radiograph shows appropriate filling of the defect with the graft.

intramedullary nailing.[8] A vast majority of cases were open fractures and one-half of their patients had evidence of infection after the index procedure. Bone marrow was aspirated from the posterior iliac crest a mean of 14.3 months from initial injury. It was obtained in small aliquots and not concentrated. The bone marrow aspirate was injected typically into the posterolateral aspect of the tibial nonunion. Additionally, the bone marrow aspirate was not the sole

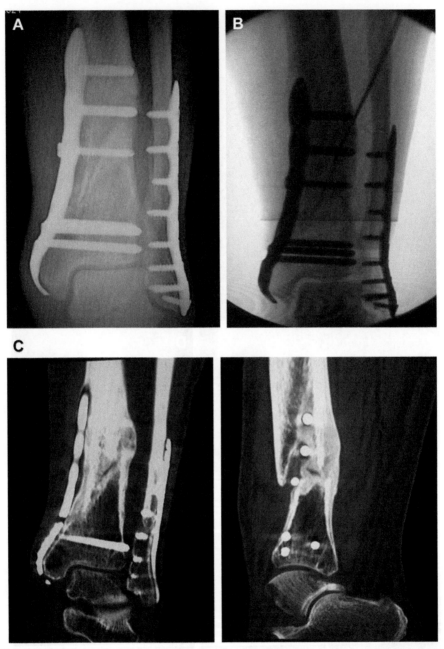

Fig. 2. (*A*) A 45-year-old woman underwent internal fixation for a distal tibia fracture at an outside institution was referred for persistent leg pain owing to a nonunion 12 months after her index procedure. Preoperative computed tomography (CT) imaging demonstrated less than 5% fracture healing. (*B*) She underwent bone marrow aspiration and percutaneous grafting. Four months after the grafting procedure, CT imaging (*C*) demonstrated greater than 50% healing and her leg pain had improved significantly. (*Courtesy of* Mark Brinker, MD, Houston, TX.)

treatment; 50% of patients had intramedullary nailing performed at the time of injection. They reported a 90% union rate (18/20) and advocated for the use of bone marrow aspirate as a viable alternative to autologous grafting.

Hernigou and colleagues[10] reported their results of 60 tibial nonunion patients treated exclusively with BMAC. The location of the nonunion was heterogenous with a majority (52%; 31/60) located within the midshaft. Additionally, 48 of the nonunions were initially open fractures and treated with external fixation. The remaining cases were closed and treated in a cast. All nonunions were considered aseptic and atrophic. BMAC was injected after a mean of 8 months from initial injury. They found that 88% of their patients obtained union with no further intervention. Similar success was reported by Braly and colleagues,[11] who described the outcome of 11 distal metadiaphyseal tibial nonunions treated exclusively with bone marrow aspirate. All 11 patients were treated initially with plates and screws and were considered to have aseptic and atrophic nonunions. The aspirate was harvested from the posterior iliac crest and it was not concentrated. The mean time from injury to bone marrow aspiration injection was 8 months. They found that 82% of patients (9/11) had successful union.

Bone marrow aspirate and BMAC injection has also been reported to treat nonunions in the femur, humerus, and ulna successfully.[14–17] One of the earliest studies, by Garg and colleagues,[14] reported their outcomes of tibial, humerus, and ulnar nonunions treated exclusively with bone marrow aspirate. They reported injecting 15 to 20 mL of posterior iliac crest bone marrow aspirate after a mean of 10 months from initial injury. They found that 85% (17/20) healed with no further intervention.

Unfortunately, no comparative studies of bone marrow aspirate injection with other nonunion treatment techniques, such as intramedullary nail dynamization, exchange nailing, or compressive plating with autologous bone grafting has been performed. However, analyzing studies with similar cohorts can extrapolate generalized comparisons between these different nonunion treatment techniques. Guimaraes and colleagues[17] recently reported their outcomes of femoral shaft nonunions that were initially treated with locked intramedullary nailing who subsequently underwent percutaneous BMAC injection. They found that 50% of patients (8/16) had successful union of their fracture. This number compares favorably to previous publications, which reported a 58% to 76% success with intramedullary nail dynamization,[18,19] and 53% to 88% success with exchange nailing.[19,20] It should be noted that the bone marrow aspirate cohort from Guimaraes and associates[17] performed their secondary procedure at a mean of 41 months after initial injury and treatment. Likewise, comparing common treatment options for tibial shaft nonunions shows that bone marrow aspirate compares favorably as well. As mentioned, tibial unions treated with bone marrow aspirate achieved union in 75% to 90% of cases,[8–12] whereas nail dynamization or exchange nailing has been found to be successful in 83% and 90% of cases, respectfully.[21] However, caution must be exercised when directly comparing the different studies as numerous unaccounted for cofounding variables and potentially dissimilar treatment groups likely exist. The point of comparing the success of the different treatment techniques is to show that equipoise exists and a large, randomized study is needed to definitively compare treatments and better delineate the nonunion characteristics for when percutaneous bone marrow aspirate injection is the most efficacious treatment option.

SURGICAL TECHNIQUE

Owing to the varied clinical scenarios often being addressed with the use of bone marrow aspiration and the lack of robust clinical trials, no standardized technique for bone marrow aspiration and grafting exists. However, multiple aspects of the procedure require specific attention to maximize efficacy and minimize clinical complications, including the location of aspiration, the neurovascular structures at risk, the size of syringe, the volume aspirated from each area, and the necessity to concentrate the aspirate. Each of these factors deserves individual consideration.

Bone Marrow Harvest Location

Bone marrow aspiration from the iliac crest is considered the gold standard location for orthopedic trauma and extremity surgery. However, controversy exists as to the best location within the iliac crest and whether other anatomic locations can provide an equivalent number or concentration of MSCs. Pierini and colleagues[22] compared the concentration of MSCs between bone marrow aspirated from the anterior and posterior iliac crests in 22 patients. They found that the mean number of MSCs from the posterior iliac crest was 60% greater than from the anterior iliac crest. This difference was significant. They concluded that harvesting bone marrow from the posterior iliac crest was preferable. Although the posterior crest may maximize the number of harvested MSCs, several factors may influence the site of bone marrow harvest, including the positioning of the patient for the subsequent grafting procedure, the inability to position the patient prone, surgeon familiarity with iliac crest anatomy, and the use of a point-of-care bone marrow concentrator.

Besides the location within the crest for bone marrow aspiration, Hyer and colleagues[23] investigated the MSC yield from different anatomic sites. Their group harvested bone marrow from the calcaneus, distal tibia, and iliac crest from the same patient. A total of 40 patients were enrolled in the study. They found that MSCs were obtained from all 3 sites, but in significantly different concentrations. The distal tibia (32.4 MSCs/mL) and calcaneus (7.1 MSCs/mL) had a 96.4% and 99.2%, respectively, lower concentration of MSCs compared with the iliac crest (898.4 MSCs/mL). This study confirmed that aspirate from the iliac crest is preferred.

Iliac Crest Osseous Anatomy

Although bone marrow aspirate from the posterior crest has been found to have the highest concentrate of MSCs, it can be harvested from any site along the crest from the anterior superior iliac spine (ASIS) to the posterior superior iliac spine. The distance from the ASIS to the posterior superior iliac spine along the iliac crest has been estimated to be approximately 24 cm.[24] Bone marrow aspiration can occur at any point along this distance. However, depending on the location, there are significant changes in the iliac wing width, which increases the potential for cortical penetration as well as alters the proximity to neurovascular structures. Hernigou and colleagues,[24] divided the length of the iliac crest into 6 different sections starting at the ASIS that were each approximately 4 cm in length. The sections were pie-shaped, with each dividing line converging at the center of the hip. The thickness between the inner and outer iliac wing cortices was calculated for each of the sections, and the ability of each section to accommodate a hypothetical 3-mm trocar was determined. They found that sections 1, 4, and 5 had the thinnest areas of ilium resulting in an increased risk of cortical penetration. They observed that sections 2 and 3 (4–12 cm posterior to the ASIS) as well as section 6 (from the posterior superior iliac spine to a point 4 cm anterior to it) are the most amenable for trocar placement given their increased iliac wing width.

Neurovascular Structures at Risk

The proximity of important neurovascular structures such as the lateral femoral cutaneous nerve, external iliac artery, sciatic nerve, and superior gluteal vessels to the iliac cortex changes depending on the location of trocar insertion. Hernigou and colleagues[25] studied 48 hemipelvic CT angiography scans to estimate whether a hypothetical 10-cm length trocar placed with up to a 20° deviation in the insertion angle could result in damage to various neurovascular

structures. Using a similar ilium dividing scheme of 6 pie-shaped sections (as described), they found that the risk to the external iliac artery was the greatest for the anterior sections. The external iliac artery was found to be within a hypothetical area of a misplaced trocar in 45.8% and 62.5% of cases for sections 1 and 2, respectively. This risk decreased substantially as the trocar insertion location was moved posteriorly to sections 3 (18.8%) and 4 (14.6%). Additionally, the authors found that the sciatic notch was located a mean of 70 mm from the iliac crest. They concluded that any trocar inserted in sections 5 and 6 to a depth of greater than 60 mm and only 5° of deviation risked cortical penetration and possible injury to the either the sciatic nerve or superior gluteal vessels.

Syringe Size

Although the size of syringe used for bone marrow aspiration seems trivial, 1 study has demonstrated that it has a significant impact on the number of obtained MSCs. Hernigou and colleagues[26] compared the MSC concentration in aspirate using a 10- or 50-mL syringe. Thirty patients had bone marrow aspiration harvest performed on both iliac wings. One side had multiple aspirations at standardized sites of different volumes using a 10-mL syringe and the other side had a similar protocol but using a 50-mL syringe. The 10-mL syringe aspirated 1-, 2-, 4-, and 10-mL volumes, whereas the 50-mL syringe aspirated 5-, 10-, 20-, and 50-mL volumes. The aspirate from each site using the 2 different syringes were then analyzed and compared. They found that the concentration of MSCs was approximately 300% higher in the 10-mL syringe cohort for similar volume aspirations. They hypothesized that if the same force is used to withdrawal the syringe plunger, the smaller diameter plunger would create a higher negative pressure (pressure = force/area) resulting in a greater MSC harvest. Their recommendation was to use a smaller volume syringe and perform aspirations at multiple sites.

Aspirate Volume

The volume of aspirate has also been found to influence the harvested MSC concentration. Muschler and colleagues[27] first studied the effect of aspiration volume by comparing 1-, 2-, and 4-mL bone marrow aspirate samples. They found that although the total number of MSCs increased with greater aspirated volumes, so did the quantity of diluting peripheral blood. The harvested MSC concentration decreased 28% (1451–1051 MSCs/mL) between 1- and

2-mL volumes and 38% (1418–882 MSCs/mL) between 2- and 4-mL aspiration volumes. They recommended limiting the aspiration volumes to less than 2 mL from 1 site unless intraoperative processing to concentrate the sample was to be used. Similar findings were reported by Hernigou and colleagues,[26] who calculated the concentration of MSCs obtained after aspirating different volumes using a similar sized syringe from a single site. They found that an increased concentration of MSCs was obtained with smaller aspirated volumes. For example, when using a 10-mL syringe, the concentration of MSCs decreased a mean of 82% from their 1- and 10-mL aspirated samples, or from 2062 MSCs/mL to 376 MSCs/mL. Their conclusion was that an aspiration of 10% to 20% of the syringe volume was ideal. With increasing aspiration volumes, they postulated that the sample may be diluted with peripheral blood thereby decreasing the MSC concentration.

Concentrating Aspirate

There is no consensus about whether the bone marrow aspirate should be concentrated. Studies have shown that BMAC has a greater concentration of MSCs than unconcentrated aspirate. Hernigou and colleagues[10] measured the concentration of MSCs in aspirate before and after concentration. In their technique, bone marrow aspirate was centrifuged to separate the heavier polynuclear cell layer, which was then isolated and analyzed. An initial aspirate volume of 300 mL was typically reduced to 60 mL after the concentrating process, and the aspirate concentration increased from 612 MSCs/mL before concentrating to 2579 MSCs/mL after concentrating. Furthermore, after injection of the BMAC into 60 tibial nonunions, they reported a significant difference in the MSC concentration and overall number of injected MSCs between the patients who subsequently achieved union and those that did not. The patients successfully treated with BMAC had a mean aspirate concentrate of 2835 MSCs/mL, whereas the persistent nonunion patients had 634 MSCs/mL. All of the patients who were unsuccessfully treated had aspirate containing less than 1000 MSCs/mL or fewer than 30,000 total MSCs injected. Age, sex, and medical comorbidities were not associated with treatment outcome. This study was instrumental in confirming that the concentration and total number of MSCs injected are 2 of the most important factors.

Although the concentration process can optimize the success of bone marrow aspirate grafting in treating nonunions, the need for additional equipment and possible increased operative time can create obstacles in implementing this step. A handful of published case series have described successful results when bone marrow aspirate concentrating was not performed.[8,9,11,14,16,28] It must be emphasized that if a concentration process is not to be used, other steps to maximize the concentration and total number of obtained MSCs should be used such as aspirating multiple small volume aliquots with small syringes as well as obtaining aspirate from the posterior iliac crest.

Clinical Complication Rate

As mentioned, there are numerous neurovascular and visceral structures potentially at risk when performing an iliac crest bone marrow aspiration. This is true whether aspirating from the anterior or posterior iliac crest. However, the reported clinical morbidity is low. Bain[29] surveyed members of the British Society of Haematology and collected information regarding the number or bone marrow biopsy procedures performed and the number of "biopsy-related misadventures." She found that of approximately 55,000 procedures, only 26 adverse events were reported, an 0.05% incidence. The most frequent adverse event was hemorrhage and one death resulted from the procedure. Other authors have also described cases of large volume hemorrhage with bone marrow biopsy or aspiration.[30,31] In the orthopedic literature, Hernigou and colleagues[32] reviewed 523 bone marrow aspiration cases over a 16-year period and compared them with a separate cohort of 435 patients who underwent a standard iliac crest bone graft harvest. These investigators found that the rate of complication with bone marrow aspiration was approximately 7.6%. Complications included patients who experienced anemia not requiring transfusion, early or persistent pain at the site of aspiration, neuralgia, hematoma or seroma formation, superficial wound infection, ossification at the aspiration site, and harvest site fracture. Of note, none of the patients required surgical treatment of the complications and all were managed successfully with observation. In comparison, summation of the same complications in the iliac crest bone graft harvest cohort revealed a significantly higher rate of 80.2%. The authors concluded that the rate of complication with bone marrow aspirate was 10 times less frequent as with standard iliac crest bone graft harvest and is a relatively safe procedure.

One other hypothetical concern with the application of bone marrow aspirate into any extremity site is the possibility of an increased cancer risk. This theoretic risk is due to the ability of pluripotent stem cells to either differentiate into or stimulate a tumorigenic process. Hernigou and colleagues[33] reviewed 1873 cases of patients treated with bone marrow aspirate to see if any tumors developed either locally or elsewhere and compared that with general population data. They found that no tumors formed at the treatment site and only 53 cancers developed elsewhere, which was lower than the incidence in the general population. They concluded that bone marrow aspirate injection did not increase a patient's propensity to develop cancer.

Technique

Phillippe Hernigou and his group from Paris, France, have the largest published case volume regarding iliac crest bone marrow aspiration. Through meticulous research analyzing and improving their techniques, they have developed several methods to obtain the highest concentrate MSC aspirate possible.[34] The typical steps of a bone marrow aspiration are as follows.

- The patient is positioned supine, lateral decubitus, or prone depending on the planned harvest site and patient position for subsequent injection.
- The affected extremity and one or both of the iliac crests are prepped and draped in the standard sterile fashion.
- A disposable or reusable trocar needle with a beveled edge (ie, Jamshidi or Lee-Lok needle; Fig. 3) is inserted through a small skin incision along the iliac crest.
- The needle is inserted either manually through the iliac crest cortex with a twisting motion or gentle malleting until it is at a depth of approximately 6 cm.
- A heparinized 10-mL syringe is attached to the back of the needle (5000 units of sodium heparin diluted in 5 mL of normal saline is run through the syringe before use to prevent coagulation of the aspirate).
- Aliquots of 2 to 4 mL are aspirated at a time with the needle being turned 45° with each aspiration as the bevel will preferentially withdrawal from that quadrant.
- Once an entire rotation has been performed, the needle is withdrawn 1 to 2 cm and the process is repeated.

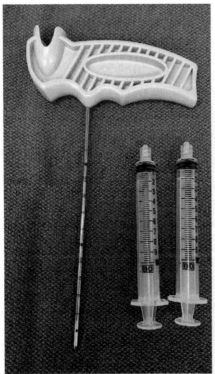 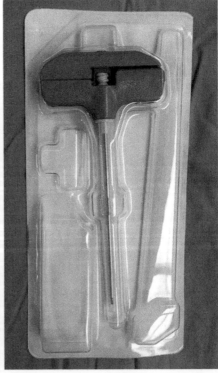

Fig. 3. Two types of commercially available disposable bone marrow aspirate needles.

- The needle is repositioned on the iliac crest approximately 2 cm from the prior insertion site and another round of multiple aspirations is performed.
- A total of 2 to 5 separate sites within 1 section of the iliac crest is typically performed depending on the amount of bone marrow needed.
- The aspirate is either used in its unprocessed state or concentrated using a commercially or institutionally owned centrifuge.
- Under orthogonal fluoroscopy, either the same aspiration needle or an 18-gauge spinal needle is inserted into the fracture site (Fig. 4).
- The site of largest osseous gap or defect should be targeted based on preoperative imaging.
- The aspirate is injected slowly, approximately 20 mL per minute, until significant resistance is felt.
- Aspirate should also be injected around the periphery of the fracture site as well (see Fig. 4).
- The total volume of aspirate injected can be between 20 and 80 mL depending on the fracture location; injected volumes as

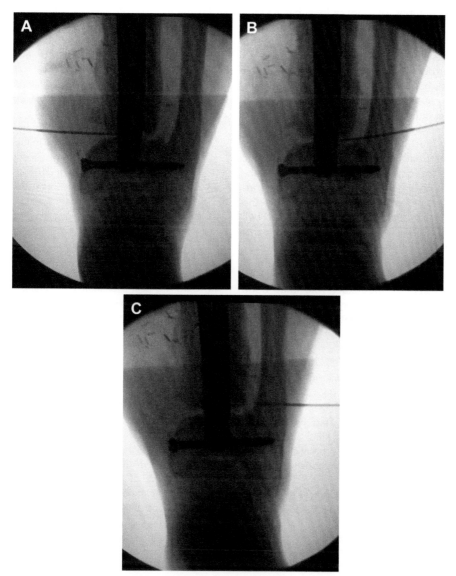

Fig. 4. Using fluoroscopic guidance to inject bone marrow aspirate directly into a nonunion site (A, B) as well as the periphery of the nonunion site (C). (*Courtesy of* Mark Brinker, MD, Houston, TX.)

high as 150 mL have been reported,[13] although great caution should be exercised with higher volumes.

- The needle is slowly removed and direct pressure is applied to the injection site.
- Postoperatively, patients are typically immobilized and weight bearing is restricted for 4 to 6 weeks to avoid mechanical disruption of the bone healing process; progressive weight bearing is initiated after that.

SUMMARY

The use of bone marrow aspirate in orthopedic trauma is still in its infancy. Although an increasing number of publications have highlighted the clinical success of using this treatment, there remains no universally accepted role for its use. The obvious advantages of bone marrow aspirate are that it is readily obtainable, has a low harvest morbidity, and is an easily and quickly performed technique when used either in combination with allograft or as a stand-alone graft to inject into a fracture. Currently, most publications have detailed its use in the treatment of aseptic and atrophic nonunions that have no significant alignment abnormalities or large fracture gap. Expanding indications for bone marrow aspirate use in the treatment of other types of nonunions as well as its use in the acute fracture setting needs to be further defined. Future studies directly comparing its use with more conventional techniques such as iliac crest autograft are needed to firmly establish the exact role that bone marrow aspirate should play in the treatment of orthopedic trauma patients.

REFERENCES

1. Hernigou P, Poignard A, Manicom O, et al. The use of percutaneous autologous bone marrow transplantation in nonunion and avascular necrosis of bone. J Bone Joint Surg Br 2005;87(7):896–902.
2. Crane JL, Cao X. Bone marrow mesenchymal stem cells and TGF-beta signaling in bone remodeling. J Clin Invest 2014;124(2):466–72.
3. Bianco P. Bone and the hematopoietic niche: a tale of two stem cells. Blood 2011;117(20):5281–8.
4. Schmidmaier G, Herrmann S, Green J, et al. Quantitative assessment of growth factors in reaming aspirate, iliac crest, and platelet preparation. Bone 2006;39(5):1156–63.
5. Gianakos A, Ni A, Zambrana L, et al. Bone marrow aspirate concentrate in animal long bone healing: an analysis of basic science evidence. J Orthop Trauma 2016;30(1):1–9.
6. Hernigou P, Dubory A, Roubineau F, et al. Allografts supercharged with bone-marrow-derived mesenchymal stem cells possess equivalent osteogenic capacity to that of autograft: a study with long-term follow-ups of human biopsies. Int Orthop 2017;41(1):127–32.
7. Jager M, Herten M, Fochtmann U, et al. Bridging the gap: bone marrow aspiration concentrate reduces autologous bone grafting in osseous defects. J Orthop Res 2011;29(2):173–80.
8. Connolly JF, Guse R, Tiedeman J, et al. Autologous marrow injection as a substitute for operative grafting of tibial nonunions. Clin Orthop Relat Res 1991;(266):259–70.
9. Goel A, Sangwan SS, Siwach RC, et al. Percutaneous bone marrow grafting for the treatment of tibial non-union. Injury 2005;36(1):203–6.
10. Hernigou P, Poignard A, Beaujean F, et al. Percutaneous autologous bone-marrow grafting for nonunions. influence of the number and concentration of progenitor cells. J Bone Joint Surg Am 2005;87(7):1430–7.
11. Braly HL, O'Connor DP, Brinker MR. Percutaneous autologous bone marrow injection in the treatment of distal meta-diaphyseal tibial nonunions and delayed unions. J Orthop Trauma 2013;27(9):527–33.
12. Desai P, Hasan SM, Zambrana L, et al. Bone mesenchymal stem cells with growth factors successfully treat nonunions and delayed unions. HSS J 2015;11(2):104–11.
13. Connolly JF, Guse R, Tiedeman J, et al. Autologous marrow injection for delayed unions of the tibia: a preliminary report. J Orthop Trauma 1989;3(4):276–82.
14. Garg NK, Gaur S, Sharma S. Percutaneous autogenous bone marrow grafting in 20 cases of ununited fracture. Acta Orthop Scand 1993;64(6):671–2.
15. Garnavos C, Mouzopoulos G, Morakis E. Fixed intramedullary nailing and percutaneous autologous concentrated bone-marrow grafting can promote bone healing in humeral-shaft fractures with delayed union. Injury 2010;41(6):563–7.
16. Kassem MS. Percutaneous autogenous bone marrow injection for delayed union or non union of fractures after internal fixation. Acta Orthop Belg 2013;79(6):711–7.
17. Guimaraes JA, Duarte ME, Fernandes MB, et al. The effect of autologous concentrated bone-marrow grafting on the healing of femoral shaft non-unions after locked intramedullary nailing. Injury 2014;45(Suppl 5):S7–13.
18. Wu CC. The effect of dynamization on slowing the healing of femur shaft fractures after interlocking nailing. J Trauma 1997;43(2):263–7.
19. Pihlajamaki HK, Salminen ST, Bostman OM. The treatment of nonunions following intramedullary

nailing of femoral shaft fractures. J Orthop Trauma 2002;16(6):394–402.

20. Weresh MJ, Hakanson R, Stover MD, et al. Failure of exchange reamed intramedullary nails for ununited femoral shaft fractures. J Orthop Trauma 2000;14(5):335–8.

21. Litrenta J, Tornetta P 3rd, Vallier H, et al. Dynamizations and exchanges: success rates and indications. J Orthop Trauma 2015;29(12):569–73.

22. Pierini M, Di Bella C, Dozza B, et al. The posterior iliac crest outperforms the anterior iliac crest when obtaining mesenchymal stem cells from bone marrow. J Bone Joint Surg Am 2013;95(12): 1101–7.

23. Hyer CF, Berlet GC, Bussewitz BW, et al. Quantitative assessment of the yield of osteoblastic connective tissue progenitors in bone marrow aspirate from the iliac crest, tibia, and calcaneus. J Bone Joint Surg Am 2013;95(14):1312–6.

24. Hernigou J, Alves A, Homma Y, et al. Anatomy of the ilium for bone marrow aspiration: map of sectors and implication for safe trocar placement. Int Orthop 2014;38(12):2585–90.

25. Hernigou J, Picard L, Alves A, et al. Understanding bone safety zones during bone marrow aspiration from the iliac crest: the sector rule. Int Orthop 2014;38(11):2377–84.

26. Hernigou P, Homma Y, Flouzat Lachaniette CH, et al. Benefits of small volume and small syringe for bone marrow aspirations of mesenchymal stem cells. Int Orthop 2013;37(11):2279–87.

27. Muschler GF, Boehm C, Easley K. Aspiration to obtain osteoblast progenitor cells from human bone marrow: the influence of aspiration volume. J Bone Joint Surg Am 1997;79(11): 1699–709.

28. Singh AK, Shetty S, Saraswathy JJ, et al. Percutaneous autologous bone marrow injections for delayed or non-union of bones. J Orthop Surg (Hong Kong) 2013;21(1):60–4.

29. Bain BJ. Bone marrow biopsy morbidity and mortality. Br J Haematol 2003;121(6):949–51.

30. Ben-Chetrit E, Flusser D, Assaf Y. Severe bleeding complicating percutaneous bone marrow biopsy. Arch Intern Med 1984;144(11):2284.

31. Tsai HL, Liu SW, How CK, et al. A rare case of massive retroperitoneal hemorrhage after bone marrow aspiration alone. Am J Emerg Med 2008; 26(9):1070.e5-6.

32. Hernigou P, Desroches A, Queinnec S, et al. Morbidity of graft harvesting versus bone marrow aspiration in cell regenerative therapy. Int Orthop 2014;38(9):1855–60.

33. Hernigou P, Homma Y, Flouzat-Lachaniette CH, et al. Cancer risk is not increased in patients treated for orthopaedic diseases with autologous bone marrow cell concentrate. J Bone Joint Surg Am 2013;95(24):2215–21.

34. Hernigou P, Mathieu G, Poignard A, et al. Percutaneous autologous bone-marrow grafting for nonunions. Surgical technique. J Bone Joint Surg Am 2006;88(Suppl 1 Pt 2):322–7.

Pediatrics

Orthobiologics in Pediatric Orthopedics

Robert F. Murphy, MD*, James F. Mooney III, MD

KEYWORDS

- Allograft • Scoliosis • Foot reconstruction • Tibia pseudarthrosis • BMP

KEY POINTS

- Use of orthobiologics in pediatric orthopedics is less frequent than in other orthopedic subspecialties.
- Allograft is effective in a variety of pediatric spinal deformity conditions in enhancing bony arthrodesis while avoiding morbidity of autograft harvest.
- Structural allograft can be used safely in foot deformity reconstruction.
- Recombinant BMP may be successful in enhancing healing of congenital pseudarthrosis of the tibia.
- The use of bioabsorable implants to stabilize children's fractures is an emerging concept.

INTRODUCTION

The types of biologic devices or products used in orthopedics to enhance or augment bone formation can be grouped broadly into 3 categories: osteoinductive, osteoconductive, and osteogenic.[1] Osteoinductive products encourage the host site to develop cells that form bone. Osteoconductive products are inert scaffolds that serve as a framework on which the host can produce bone. Osteogenic products are capable of independently producing bone-forming cells.

In adult orthopedics, reports of the use of orthobiologics are numerous, especially in the fields of orthopedic trauma,[2] adult spine surgery,[3] and foot and ankle surgery.[4] However, reports on the use of biologics in pediatric orthopedics are less common.[5] This may be due to the greater healing potential and more predictable bone formation in children compared with adults. Furthermore, children have fewer known comorbidities associated with deficiencies in bone healing in adults, including cigarette smoking, diabetes, and cardiovascular disease.

In pediatric orthopedics, most clinical applications of orthobiologics involve osteoconductive materials. These products are usually autograft substitutes, used in either a structural or augmentative fashion. A major benefit to the use of autograft substitutes is the elimination of the morbidity of an autograft harvest.[6–8] Limited reports exist regarding the use of osteoinductive substances, such as bone morphogenic proteins, in pediatric orthopedic patients. The clinical applications of osteogenic substances in pediatric orthopedics is limited primarily to injection of autologous bone marrow aspirate to treat unicameral bone cysts[9,10] or to stimulate bone formation in other lytic benign tumorous conditions.[11] To date, the use of other osteogenic substances, such as platelet-rich plasma, has undergone little formal evaluation in pediatric orthopedic patients.

SPINE

Scoliosis, whether adolescent, congenital, or neuromuscular, is a common condition treated by pediatric orthopedic surgeons. In patients with deformities of sufficient magnitude that

---

Disclosure Statement: No relevant disclosures to this article.
Department of Orthopaedics, Medical University of South Carolina, 96 Jonathan Lucas Street, CSB 708, Charleston, SC 29492, USA
* Corresponding author.
E-mail address: murphyr@musc.edu

Orthop Clin N Am 48 (2017) 323–331
http://dx.doi.org/10.1016/j.ocl.2017.03.007
0030-5898/17/© 2017 Elsevier Inc. All rights reserved.

demonstrate progression, or are at risk of progression, spinal fusion with instrumentation may be indicated. The goals of surgery are to obtain a solid arthrodesis, so as to prevent later curve progression, and correct the deformity to the degree that is safely possible.

Idiopathic and Neuromuscular Scoliosis

From the earliest reports, spinal fusion procedures for scoliosis were augmented with autograft, most commonly harvested from the posterior iliac crest.[12] Autograft was considered to be essential to minimize the risks of pseudarthrosis and curve progression in the setting of uninstrumented fusions and early generation instrumentation systems.[13] However, harvest of autogenous posterior iliac crest bone graft is not a benign procedure[6,7] and can be associated with complications, including pain and/or local neuropraxia, that may be severe enough to interfere with activities of daily living.[8] These issues have led surgeons to evaluate alternatives that would still augment the body's natural mechanisms in generating a solid bony arthrodesis without incurring the risks of autogenous graft harvest. Orthobiologic products that have been investigated include freeze-dried allograft, synthetic ceramic bone substitutes, and allograft supplemented with bone marrow aspirate.

Following the development of modern segmental spinal instrumentation, early reports were encouraging that allograft could be used safely, with acceptable fusion rates and limited evidence of pseudarthrosis[14–17] (Fig. 1). Other investigators found that isolated allograft was not as successful but, by adding bone marrow aspirate, fusion rates similar to those reported with autograft could be achieved.[18] Still others found satisfactory arthrodesis rates using a synthetic porous ceramic product.[19,20] Long-term 5-year minimum follow-up on subjects treated with allograft showed a pseudarthrosis rate of 2.7% and loss of correction of 5.9%.[21]

One of the foremost concerns regarding allograft use is the potential for infection. Although some data exist that demonstrates increased rates of surgical site infections following use of allograft,[22,23] other reports refute this claim.[24,25] In 2 separate prospective randomized trials of spinal fusion in idiopathic scoliosis subjects,[19,20] synthetic ceramic was found to produce equal rates of fusion, with no increase rate of infection. To date, no similar studies exist that compare allograft with autograft.

Additional considerations regarding risk of infection in pediatric spine surgery concern the addition of antibiotics to any graft substance.

The addition of gentamicin to bone graft has been shown to decrease rates of postoperative surgical site infection in cerebral palsy patients undergoing spinal fusion with unit rod instrumentation.[26] No further data exist regarding indications for antibiotic use in children undergoing spinal fusion surgery. The choice of antibiotic, as well as dose and location of use (either in the local wound bed or within a graft substance), must be tailored to each clinical situation. In a consensus statement regarding best practice guidelines in pediatric spine surgery, addition of antibiotic within the surgical site was recommended in high risk cases.[27]

Other Spine

The use of allograft has been reported in other spine applications besides idiopathic and neuromuscular scoliosis. Traditionally, allograft use has been discouraged in the cervical spine due to historical studies reporting near universal failure.[28] In 2015, Reintjes and colleagues[29] published a meta-analysis that assessed the use of allograft and autograft in association with pediatric patients undergoing posterior cervical fusion or occipitocervical fusion. They found a statistically higher fusion rate with use of autograft and in fusions that included the occiput. However, the investigators noted a wide variability in fixation systems and the use of other osteoinductive agents. To date, there are no studies that compare long-term fusion rates between allograft and autograft using comparable implant and instrumentation systems.

Although autograft is still recommended at the occipitocervical junction, more recent data show that allograft can be used successfully in the pediatric subaxial cervical spine. Murphy and colleagues[30] reported on 26 subjects who underwent rigid segmental spinal instrumentation and allograft or autograft for a variety of conditions and disorders in the subaxial cervical spine. When compared with allograft, autograft subjects had similar rates of fusion with acceptable rates of complications. Given the ability to avoid donor site morbidity,[8] the investigators recommended consideration of allograft in cases of subaxial pediatric cervical spine fusion with rigid segmental spinal instrumentation. In a review of 107 subjects with congenital spine deformity, Hedequist and colleagues[31] reported a 97% union rate when using freeze-dried corticocancellous graft and instrumentation, with few complications.

There has been increasing information regarding the use of bone morphogenetic protein (BMP) in pediatric spinal deformity patients.

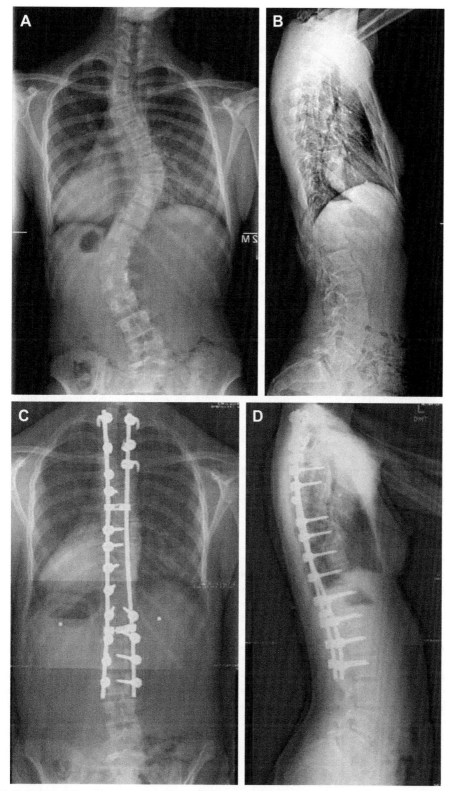

Fig. 1. (A, B) Preoperative posteroanterior (PA) and lateral radiographs of a 16-year-old girl with adolescent idiopathic scoliosis and a progressive deformity. She underwent posterior spinal fusion with segmental instrumentation and allograft augmentation. (C, D) Six-month postoperative PA and lateral radiographs demonstrate deformity correction with satisfactory evidence of fusion with no apparent complications.

To date, the use of BMP in pediatric patients is considered off-label for all indications by the US Food and Drug Administration. There have been concerns regarding increased complication rates in adult spinal fusion patients. In 2013, Carragee and colleagues[32] reported an increased risk of new cancer in adult patients undergoing lumbar spinal arthrodesis procedures using BMP. However, since that time, further large cohorts of adult patients undergoing lumbar arthrodesis showed no evidence of increased cancer risk with utilization of BMP.[33]

Reports of BMP use in pediatric spinal fusion procedures have become more frequent. Rocque and colleagues[34] reviewed information on 4658 pediatric spinal fusion subjects available through a private payer database. Of these, 93.1% underwent a thoracolumbar fusion and BMP was used in 37.6% of all spinal fusion subjects in this cohort. The investigators found no difference in acute complications between the BMP and non-BMP groups. In 2015, Sayama and colleagues[35] reviewed 57 consecutive posterior spinal fusion subjects treated with BMP with a minimum of 24 months follow-up. They found no new cases of cancer or spread of any existing malignancies in this subject group.

Most recently, Garg and colleagues[36] performed a retrospective review of 312 subjects from 5 medical centers who underwent BMP application as part of an orthopedic procedure from 2000 to 2013. Of the 312 subjects, 228 (73%) underwent a spinal fusion procedure. In subjects treated with BMP, 22% were noted to have had a major or minor complication. Infection and implant failures were the most common major complication.

Overall, it seems that there is some role for the use of BMP application in pediatric spinal surgery, particularly in the face of deformity or nonunion. Complication rates are similar in patients with and without BMP utilization, at least in the short term, and the concern about increased cancer risk has not been shown in pediatric patients to date. However, significant questions remain as to the indications and patient population that will be best served by the use of this specific orthobiologic agent in pediatric spinal patients.

FOOT AND ANKLE

Foot reconstructions in patients with symptomatic planovalgus or cavovarus feet that fail nonoperative management are common in many pediatric orthopedic practices. In many of these procedures, bone graft is required to obtain and maintain the position of the newly corrected foot. As in other areas in orthopedics, structural autograft is the gold standard, due to strength, nonimmunogenicity, and ease of incorporation. However, as noted previously, iliac crest autograft harvest and utilization is not without potential complications.[8]

Fresh frozen structural allograft has been used most commonly, and studied most frequently, in pediatric foot and ankle procedures, particularly in the management of pes planovalgus deformity with calcaneal lengthening osteotomy. In his original report detailing lateral column lengthening with a modified Evans osteotomy, Mosca[37] used tricortical iliac allograft in 13 of 20 subjects, with an acceptable rate of complications and avoidance of donor site morbidity (Fig. 2). In a larger follow-up series of 161 children who had foot reconstruction, with the use of 182 allografts and 63 autografts, Vining and colleagues[38] reported similar rates of incorporation between allograft and autograft. All cases of allograft failure were attributed to technical error, rather than graft type. Furthermore, these investigators found that when accounting for iliac crest operating room harvest time, as well as surgeon fees for graft harvest, use of allograft resulted in a savings of approximately 25% per case. Other investigators have also reported successful use of structural allograft in pediatric foot reconstruction surgery, with acceptable rates of complications.[39]

Ledford and colleagues[40] reported on the use of bovine xenograft in pediatric foot reconstruction. These investigators found an unacceptable rate of complications with a high rate of failure of graft incorporation, which led the investigators to recommend against further use.

PELVIS

In patients with developmental dysplasia of the hip and acetabular dysplasia, the Pemberton pericapsular acetabuloplasty is used by some surgeons to improve acetabular deficiency and femoral head coverage. Traditionally, autograft has been used to stabilize the osteotomy, either from the proximal femur or locally from the pelvis. However, problems with use of autograft can include availability, difficulty in obtaining appropriate graft dimensions, and graft stability.[41,42] In an attempt to limit these issues, Kessler and colleagues[43] reported on their experience using patellar allograft with a resorbable fixation pin in 26 Pemberton osteotomies. They found all osteotomies united within 3 months, the acetabular index improved from 33° to 18°.

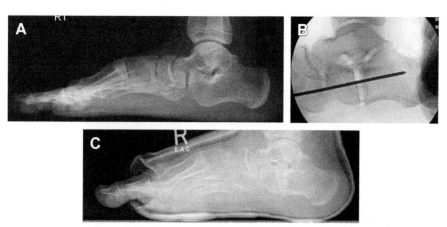

Fig. 2. (A) A 16-year-old boy with painful pes planovalgus deformity that was recalcitrant to prolonged conserva-tive management. (B) He underwent a lateral column lengthening with use of tricortical iliac crest allograft and tem-porary Kirschner wire fixation. (C) At 2 months postoperatively, he demonstrated maintenance of correction with early evidence of graft incorporation and no evidence of graft subsidence.

McCarthy and colleagues[44] compared the use of allograft to autograft in a series of 29 chil-dren and found that allograft stabilization of the osteotomy provided equal or better results, with 93% of subjects having a successful result (Fig. 3). They concluded that allograft is a viable alternative to autograft for these procedures, particularly in children with neuromuscular

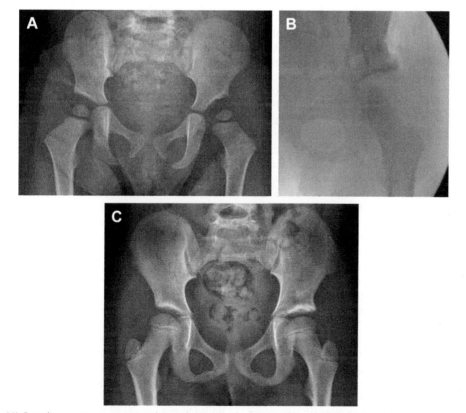

Fig. 3. (A) Standing anteroposterior pelvis radiograph of a 3-year-old girl with residual left acetabular dysplasia after undergoing successful closed reduction of left developmental dysplasia of the hip at age 6 months. (B) Intra-operative fluoroscopic image demonstrates obtaining normal horizontal position of the sourcil following Dega ace-tabuloplasty and insertion of tricortical iliac crest allograft. (C) At 3 years postoperatively, the graft has been completely incorporated with a normal appearing hip.

disorders. Other investigators have reported on the use of xenograft (calf rib) to stabilize the Pemberton osteotomy but these results are limited and have not been reproduced.[45]

TIBIA

Congenital pseudarthrosis of the tibia, often associated with neurofibromatosis, is a condition that continues to challenge pediatric orthopedic surgeons. Poor bone quality coupled with abnormally limited local vascularity make this condition particularly troublesome to treat, often requiring multiple surgeries to obtain bony union. In recalcitrant cases, persistent nonunion, pain, and/or deformity may lead to eventual amputation. The mainstay of initial surgical treatment of this condition has included the use of autologous bone graft, supplemented with either internal or external fixation.[46,47]

Recent studies have evaluated the use of recombinant human (rhBMP) in subjects undergoing surgical treatment of congenital pseudarthrosis of the tibia. Lee and colleagues[48] reviewed 5 subjects whose pseudarthrosis management was augmented by use of rhBMP-7. These investigators reported successful union in only 1 subject but noted that the use of static rigid external fixation in the treatment of these subjects may have hindered the healing potential. Other investigators, including Fabeck and colleagues,[49] have used rhBMP-7 coupled with internal fixation to achieve union. Richards and colleagues[50] reported their results regarding rhBMP-2 use with intramedullary stabilization of pseudarthrosis of the tibia. They noted union in 6 of 7 subjects treated, with no adverse events associated with the use of rhBMP-2. Spiro and colleagues[51] corroborated these results in a group of 5 subjects, who all went on to union. Four of the subjects in their series received Ilizarov external fixation in addition to rhBMP-2. In a larger retrospective series of 21 subjects, Richards and Anderson[52] reported on the use of rhBMP-2 to augment intramedullary stabilization and autograft. They demonstrated clinical and radiographic union in 16 (76%) subjects.

As noted previously regarding spinal surgery, the use of any subtype of rhBMP in the surgical management of congenital pseudarthrosis of the tibia, or in any pediatric patient, is designated off-label by the US Food and Drug Administration and little data exist on the safety of this device in skeletally immature patients. Oetgen and Richards[53] reviewed 81 surgical procedures for a diverse group of diagnoses in which rhBMP-2 was used in children and

reported a total of 16 complications. However, there was no incidence of systemic toxicity, and only 1 complication was thought to be attributable directly to the use of rhBMP-2. This was a subject with congenital kyphoscoliosis who underwent a vertebral column resection, and rhBMP-2 was used to improve fusion after deformity correction. Eleven months postoperatively, the subject presented with progressive motor weakness and MRI revealed dural fibrosis causing cord compression.

BIOABSORBABLE IMPLANTS

Metallic implants, generally stainless steel or titanium, are used in pediatric orthopedics to stabilize fractures and to maintain reduction or alignment during the healing process. Depending on the fracture location and clinical situation, metallic implants may be left protruding externally so as to facilitate removal in the clinic setting, or may be left deep to the skin. In cases of buried implants in pediatric patients, implant removal is often recommended. This requires a return to the operating room with the attendant surgical risks and potential financial implications of any operative procedure. In an effort to eliminate surgical intervention for implant removal, several bioabsorbable implants have been developed for a variety of orthopedic indications. Although their use is more common in a variety of arenas in adult orthopedics,[54–57] use of bioabsorbable implants remains relatively uncommon in children.

In a case series of 3 children, Sinikumpu and colleagues[58] used bioabsorbable intramedullary nails to stabilize radius and ulnar shaft fractures. All fractures went on to union and no implant removal was required. Fuller and colleagues[59] used bioabsorbable pins in the fixation of delayed presentation radial neck fractures in 7 children. They demonstrated no evidence of hardware irritation or need for implant removal. Podeszwa and colleagues[60] compared the use of standard metallic implants and bioabsorbable fixation methods in the management of distal tibial epiphyseal fractures. They found no increase in operative time, unplanned second surgeries, or other complications between the 2 groups. This was a retrospective analysis and the investigators concluded that there were no significant differences in the results of the use of the 2 methods but that larger prospective studies were needed. Further data on bioabsorbable implants will be necessary before widespread use becomes commonplace.

SUMMARY

Although not used as frequently as in adult orthopedics, orthobiologics serve an effective role in the treatment of certain musculoskeletal disorders in children. Allograft seems to safely augment segmental spinal instrumentation and to reliably achieve fusion in children with a variety of spinal disorders. Structural allograft can be used successfully in a variety of foot and pelvic osteotomies in children, and can eliminate the morbidity of autograft harvest. rhBMP may prove to be a valuable adjuvant in obtaining union in patients with congenital pseudarthrosis of the tibia and in some types of spinal deformity procedures. Applications of bioabsorbable implants in pediatric orthopedic trauma and deformity correction remain limited at this time.

Regarding future directions, applications of orthobiologics in pediatric orthopedics remain somewhat limited. The robust healing potential of children compared with that of adults obviates fusion enhancement in most cases. It has been shown that allograft can be used effectively in many anatomic areas in children. This efficacy will continue to limit the need for obtaining autograft and will limit the inherent risk of additional intraoperative and postoperative complications. Orthobiologic agents such as BMP may be best reserved for specific diagnoses that have proven difficult to manage successfully using existing method. Longer term complication and safety data will be necessary before making final judgments on these devices.

REFERENCES

1. Finkemeier CG. Bone-grafting and bone-graft substitutes. J Bone Joint Surg Am 2002;84A: 454–64.
2. De Long WG Jr, Einhorn TA, Koval K, et al. Bone grafts and bone graft substitutes in orthopaedic trauma surgery. A critical analysis. J Bone Joint Surg Am 2007;89:649–58.
3. Kannan A, Dodwad SN, Hsu WK. Biologics in spine arthrodesis. J Spinal Disord Tech 2015;28: 163–70.
4. Fitzgibbons TC, Hawks MA, McMullen ST, et al. Bone grafting in surgery about the foot and ankle: indications and techniques. J Am Acad Orthop Surg 2011;19:112–20.
5. Gross RH. The use of bone grafts and bone graft substitutes in pediatric orthopaedics: an overview. J Pediatr Orthop 2012;32:100–5.
6. Seiler JG 3rd, Johnson J. Iliac crest autogenous bone grafting: donor site complications. J South Orthop Assoc 2000;9:91–7.
7. Hill NM, Horne JG, Devane PA. Donor site morbidity in the iliac crest bone graft. Aust N Z J Surg 1999;69:726–8.
8. Skaggs DL, Samuelson MA, Hale JM, et al. Complications of posterior iliac crest bone grafting in spine surgery in children. Spine 2000;25:2400–2.
9. Rougraff BT, Kling TJ. Treatment of active unicameral bone cysts with percutaneous injection of demineralized bone matrix and autogenous bone marrow. J Bone Joint Surg Am 2002;84A:921–9.
10. Di Bella C, Dozza B, Frisoni T, et al. Injection of demineralized bone matrix with bone marrow concentrate improves healing in unicameral bone cyst. Clin Orthop Relat Res 2010;468:3047–55.
11. Wientroub S, Goodwin D, Khermosh O, et al. The clinical use of autologous marrow to improve osteogenic potential of bone grafts in pediatric orthopedics. J Pediatr Orthop 1989;9:186–90.
12. Moe JH. A critical analysis of methods of fusion for scoliosis; an evaluation in two hundred and sixty-six patients. J Bone Joint Surg Am 1958;40A(3):529–54. passim.
13. McMaster MJ. Stability of the scoliotic spine after fusion. J Bone Joint Surg Br 1980;62B:59–64.
14. Blanco JS, Sears CJ. Allograft bone use during instrumentation and fusion in the treatment of adolescent idiopathic scoliosis. Spine 1997;22:1338–42.
15. Jones KC, Andrish J, Kuivila T, et al. Radiographic outcomes using freeze-dried cancellous allograft bone for posterior spinal fusion in pediatric idiopathic scoliosis. J Pediatr Orthop 2002; 22.285–9.
16. Stricker SJ, Sher JS. Freeze-dried cortical allograft in posterior spinal arthrodesis: use with segmental instrumentation for idiopathic adolescent scoliosis. Orthopedics 1997;20:1039–43.
17. Grogan DP, Kalen V, Ross TI, et al. Use of allograft bone for posterior spinal fusion in idiopathic scoliosis. Clin Orthop Relat Res 1999;273–8.
18. Price CT, Connolly JF, Carantzas AC, et al. Comparison of bone grafts for posterior spinal fusion in adolescent idiopathic scoliosis. Spine 2003;28: 793–8.
19. Delecrin J, Takahashi S, Gouin F, et al. A synthetic porous ceramic as a bone graft substitute in the surgical management of scoliosis: a prospective, randomized study. Spine 2000;25:563–9.
20. Ransford AO, Morley T, Edgar MA, et al. Synthetic porous ceramic compared with autograft in scoliosis surgery. A prospective, randomized study of 341 patients. J Bone Joint Surg Br 1998;80:13–8.
21. Knapp DR Jr, Jones ET, Blanco JS, et al. Allograft bone in spinal fusion for adolescent idiopathic scoliosis. J Spinal Disord Tech 2005;(18 Suppl): S73–6.
22. Aleissa S, Parsons D, Grant J, et al. Deep wound infection following pediatric scoliosis

surgery: incidence and analysis of risk factors. Can J Surg 2011;54:263–9.

23. Sponseller PD, LaPorte DM, Hungerford MW, et al. Deep wound infections after neuromuscular scoliosis surgery: a multicenter study of risk factors and treatment outcomes. Spine 2000;25:2461–6.

24. Mikhael MM, Huddleston PM, Nassr A. Postoperative culture positive surgical site infections after the use of irradiated allograft, nonirradiated allograft, or autograft for spinal fusion. Spine 2009;34:2466–8.

25. McCarthy RE, Peek RD, Morrissy RT, et al. Allograft bone in spinal fusion for paralytic scoliosis. J Bone Joint Surg Am 1986;68:370–5.

26. Borkhuu B, Borowski A, Shah SA, et al. Antibiotic-loaded allograft decreases the rate of acute deep wound infection after spinal fusion in cerebral palsy. Spine 2008;33:2300–4.

27. Vitale MG, Riedel MD, Glotzbecker MP, et al. Building consensus: development of a Best Practice Guideline (BPG) for surgical site infection (SSI) prevention in high-risk pediatric spine surgery. J Pediatr Orthop 2013;33:471–8.

28. Stabler CL, Eismont FJ, Brown MD, et al. Failure of posterior cervical fusions using cadaveric bone graft in children. J Bone Joint Surg Am 1985;67: 371–5.

29. Reintjes SL, Amankwah EK, Rodriguez LF, et al. Allograft versus autograft for pediatric posterior cervical and occipito-cervical fusion: a systematic review of factors affecting fusion rates. J Neurosurg Pediatr 2015;1–16.

30. Murphy RF, Glotzbecker MP, Hresko MT, et al. Allograft bone use in pediatric subaxial cervical spine fusions. J Pediatr Orthop 2017;37(2):e140–4.

31. Hedequist D, Yeon H, Emans J. The use of allograft as a bone graft substitute in patients with congenital spine deformities. J Pediatr Orthop 2007;27: 686–9.

32. Carragee EJ, Chu G, Rohatgi R, et al. Cancer risk after use of recombinant bone morphogenetic protein-2 for spinal arthrodesis. J Bone Joint Surg Am 2013;95:1537–45.

33. Beachler DC, Yanik EL, Martin BI, et al. Bone morphogenetic protein use and cancer risk among patients undergoing lumbar arthrodesis: a case-cohort study using the SEER-Medicare database. J Bone Joint Surg Am 2016;98:1064–72.

34. Rocque BG, Kelly MP, Miller JH, et al. Bone morphogenetic protein-associated complications in pediatric spinal fusion in the early postoperative period: an analysis of 4658 patients and review of the literature. J Neurosurg Pediatr 2014;14:635–43.

35. Sayama C, Willsey M, Chintagumpala M, et al. Routine use of recombinant human bone morphogenetic protein-2 in posterior fusions of the pediatric spine and incidence of cancer. J Neurosurg Pediatr 2015;16:4–13.

36. Garg S, McCarthy JJ, Goodwin R, et al. Complication rates after bone morphogenetic protein (BMP) use in orthopaedic surgery in children: a concise multicenter retrospective cohort study. J Pediatr Orthop 2016. [Epub ahead of print].

37. Mosca VS. Calcaneal lengthening for valgus deformity of the hindfoot. Results in children who had severe, symptomatic flatfoot and skewfoot. J Bone Joint Surg Am 1995;77:500–12.

38. Vining NC, Warme WJ, Mosca VS. Comparison of structural bone autografts and allografts in pediatric foot surgery. J Pediatr Orthop 2012;32:719–23.

39. Nowicki PD, Tylkowski CM, Iwinski HJ, et al. Structural bone allograft in pediatric foot surgery. Am J Orthop (Belle Mead NJ) 2010;39:238–40.

40. Ledford CK, Nunley JA 2nd, Viens NA, et al. Bovine xenograft failures in pediatric foot reconstructive surgery. J Pediatr Orthop 2013;33:458–63.

41. Pemberton PA. Pericapsular osteotomy of the ilium for treatment of congenital subluxation and dislocation of the hip. J Bone Joint Surg Am 1965;47: 65–86.

42. Vedantam R, Capelli AM, Schoenecker PL. Pemberton osteotomy for the treatment of developmental dysplasia of the hip in older children. J Pediatr Orthop 1998;18:254–8.

43. Kessler JI, Stevens PM, Smith JT, et al. Use of allografts in pemberton osteotomies. J Pediatr Orthop 2001;21:468–73.

44. McCarthy JJ, Palma DA, Betz RR. Comparison of autograft and allograft fixation in Pemberton osteotomy. Orthopedics 2008;31:126.

45. Donati D, Gagliardi S, Capanna R. The use of xenograft in young patients treated with Pemberton-Zanoli osteotomy [In Italian]. Chir Organi Mov 1990;75:59–65.

46. Dobbs MB, Rich MM, Gordon JE, et al. Use of an intramedullary rod for the treatment of congenital pseudarthrosis of the tibia. Surgical technique. J Bone Joint Surg Am 2005;87(Suppl 1):33–40.

47. Dobbs MB, Rich MM, Gordon JE, et al. Use of an intramedullary rod for treatment of congenital pseudarthrosis of the tibia. A long-term follow-up study. J Bone Joint Surg Am 2004;86A:1186–97.

48. Lee FY, Sinicropi SM, Lee FS, et al. Treatment of congenital pseudarthrosis of the tibia with recombinant human bone morphogenetic protein-7 (rhBMP-7). A report of five cases. J Bone Joint Surg Am 2006;88:627–33.

49. Fabeck L, Ghafil D, Gerroudj M, et al. Bone morphogenetic protein 7 in the treatment of congenital pseudarthrosis of the tibia. J Bone Joint Surg Br 2006;88:116–8.

50. Richards BS, Oetgen ME, Johnston CE. The use of rhBMP-2 for the treatment of congenital pseudarthrosis of the tibia: a case series. J Bone Joint Surg Am 2010;92:177–85.

51. Spiro AS, Babin K, Lipovac S, et al. Combined treatment of congenital pseudarthrosis of the tibia, including recombinant human bone morphogenetic protein-2: a case series. J Bone Joint Surg Br 2011;93:695–9.

52. Richards BS, Anderson TD. rhBMP-2 and intramedullary fixation in congenital pseudarthrosis of the tibia. J Pediatr Orthop 2016. [Epub ahead of print].

53. Oetgen ME, Richards BS. Complications associated with the use of bone morphogenetic protein in pediatric patients. J Pediatr Orthop 2010;30:192–8.

54. Morandi A, Ungaro E, Fraccia A, et al. Chevron osteotomy of the first metatarsal stabilized with an absorbable pin: our 5-year experience. Foot Ankle Int 2013;34:380–5.

55. Sakai A, Oshige T, Zenke Y, et al. Mechanical comparison of novel bioabsorbable plates with titanium plates and small-series clinical comparisons for metacarpal fractures. J Bone Joint Surg Am 2012; 94:1597–604.

56. Bassuener SR, Mullis BH, Harrison RK, et al. Use of bioabsorbable pins in surgical fixation of comminuted periarticular fractures. J Orthop Trauma 2012;26:607–10.

57. Ahmad J, Jones K. Randomized, prospective comparison of bioabsorbable and steel screw fixation of lisfranc injuries. J Orthop Trauma 2016;30(12): 676–81.

58. Sinikumpu JJ, Keranen J, Haltia AM, et al. A new mini-invasive technique in treating pediatric diaphyseal forearm fractures by bioabsorbable elastic stable intramedullary nailing: a preliminary technical report. Scand J Surg 2013;102(4):258–64.

59. Fuller CB, Guillen PT, Wongworawat MD, et al. Bioabsorbable pin fixation in late presenting pediatric radial neck fractures. J Pediatr Orthop 2016;36(8): 793–6.

60. Podeszwa DA, Wilson PL, Holland AR, et al. Comparison of bioabsorbable versus metallic implant fixation for physeal and epiphyseal fractures of the distal tibia. J Pediatr Orthop 2008;28:859–63.

Orthobiologics in Pediatric Sports Medicine

Christopher C. Bray, MD[a,b,*], Clark M. Walker, MD[c], David D. Spence, MD[d]

KEYWORDS

- Orthobiologics • Pediatric sports medicine • Bone grafting • Platelet-rich protein (PRP)
- Anterior cruciate ligament (ACL) • Osteochondral defect (OCD)

KEY POINTS

- Orthobiologics are biological substances that allow injured muscles, tendons, ligaments and bone to heal more quickly. Orthobiologics stimulate healing with a variety of osteoconductive, osteoinductive, and/or osteogenic properties.
- There is a paucity of literature involving pediatric patients; however, studies are underway with potentially transferrable results indicating their use in children.
- Autograft is the primary graft choice in most pediatric cases, including ligament reconstructions and osteochondral defects.
- Plasma-rich protein has shown promise in treating tendonopathies in adults and is used as an adjunct in other sports procedures. No specific pediatric studies have been conducted.
- The future of orthobiologics in pediatric sports medicine is promising, but more investigation must be done before its routine use in pediatric sports medicine.

INTRODUCTION

Orthobiologics are biological substances that allow injured muscles, tendons, ligaments, and bones to heal more quickly. These substances occur naturally in the body and, at higher concentrations, can aid in the healing process.[1] Autograft bone, allograft bone, demineralized bone matrix, autologous bone marrow aspirate, bone morphogenic protein (BMP), platelet-rich plasma (PRP), and ceramic grafts are all types of orthobiologics.[2] Over the last 2 decades, both surgeon interest and industry development have substantially increased. A PubMed search on "orthobiologics" resulted in 66 articles dating back to 2004. In 2013, the global orthobiologics market was estimated to be $3.7 billion dollars. It is expected to increase to $5.8 billion dollars by 2018.[3] Much of the market interest is distributed throughout the subspecialties in orthopedic surgery, including trauma, foot and ankle, spine, sports medicine, and pediatrics. Their use in sports medicine has exploded in efforts to increase graft incorporation, stimulate healing, and get athletes with problems such as anterior cruciate ligament (ACL) ruptures, tendinopathies, and cartilage injuries back to sport. Because of the healing and regenerative potential in pediatric patients, there is a paucity of studies involving the use of orthobiologics in children with sports injuries. Much of their use in children has involved spinal surgery, tibial pseudarthrosis, and benign bone lesions.[2,4] The purpose of this article is to review orthobiologics and their applications in pediatric sports medicine.

Disclosure Statement: D.D. Spence, receives publishing royalties, financial or material from Elsevier.

[a] Pediatric Orthopaedic Surgery and Adolescent Sports Medicine, Department of Orthopaedic Surgery, Steadman Hawkins Clinic of the Carolinas, Greenville Health System, 701 Grove Road, Greenville, SC 29605, USA; [b] University of South Carolina School of Medicine – Greenville, Greenville, SC, USA; [c] Department of Orthopaedic Surgery, Greenville Health System, 701 Grove Road, Greenville, SC 29605, USA; [d] Department of Orthopaedic Surgery, University of Tennessee – Campbell Clinic, 1400 South Germantown Road, Germantown, Memphis, TN 38138, USA

* Corresponding author. Department of Orthopaedic Surgery, Greenville Health System, 701 Grove Road, Greenville, SC 29605.

E-mail address: cbray@ghs.org

PROPERTIES OF ORTHOBIOLOGICS

Three fundamental principles frequently are cited in describing the biology of bone grafting. All options provide unique combinations of osteoconductive, osteoinductive, and osteogenic properties (Table 1).[2,5–8]

Osteoconduction is the passive process by which a scaffold or trellis is implanted, allowing ingrowth of host capillaries, perivascular tissue, and mesenchymal stem cells (MSCs) to support ingrowth of new bone.[7,8] These osteoconductive scaffolds have structures similar to cancellous bone.[7,9] Bone autograft and allograft, demineralized bone matrix, calcium sulfate, and calcium phosphate are primary examples of osteoconductive grafts.

Osteoinduction is the process by which substances within the graft recruit pluripotent MSCs, which differentiate into osteoblasts and chondroblasts to form new bone through endosteal ossification.[5,7,8] Growth factors such as BMP, platelet-derived growth factor, interleukins, fibroblast growth factor, and vascular endothelial growth factor play a role in mediating this process. Examples of orthobiologics with osteoinductive properties include bone autograft, BMP, bone marrow aspirate, and PRP.

Osteogenesis is the synthesis of new bone from graft containing viable donor osteoblasts or their precursors. This process then promotes primary bone formation in the proper environment using MSCs, osteoblasts, and osteocytes. Fresh autologous grafts and bone marrow aspirate are orthobiologics with osteogenic properties.[5,7,8]

AUTOGRAFTS

Autologous grafting is the process by which bone and tissue are harvested from 1 site on the host and transplanted to another site in the same patient. It confers osteoconductive, osteoinductive, and osteogenic properties and is completely histocompatible. For these reasons, it is considered the "gold standard" to which all other orthobiologics are compared.[7] Autologous grafts, however, do have limitations. Donor site pain, increased blood loss, increased operative time, and the potential for donor site infection are all drawbacks. Furthermore, there is a limited supply from the host, particularly in pediatric patients.[2,7] Autologous grafts can be cortical, cancellous, or osteochondral, and include soft tissue components. Each graft varies in their biologic properties and rates and methods of incorporation. This is the predominant graft choice for most pediatric patients undergoing sports related procedures (Fig. 1).

ALLOGRAFTS

Allograft is a graft that is harvested from human cadavers, sterilely processed, and transplanted to a recipient. It can be cortical, cancellous, osteochondral, or formed into a highly processed derivative, such as demineralized bone matrix.[7] It is primarily osteoconductive, but, depending on the processing, may retain some osteoinductive properties. To prepare allograft, the soft tissues and cells are removed with ethanol and the graft is gamma irradiated for sterilization. This sterilization process adversely effects the biologic properties of the graft and

Table 1
Types of orthobiologics and their unique combinations of osteoconductive, osteoinductive, and osteogenic properties

	Osteoconductive	Osteoinductive	Osteogenic
Cortical autograft	+	+	+
Cancellous autograft	+++	+++	+++
Cortical allograft	+	+/−	−
Cancellous allograft	+	+/−	−
Demineralized bone matrix	+	++	−
Bone marrow aspirate	−	++	+++
Bone morphogenic protein	−	+	+
Plasma rich protein	−	+++	+
Ceramics	+	−	−

+, activity; −, no activity; +/−, activity depends on the preparation process.

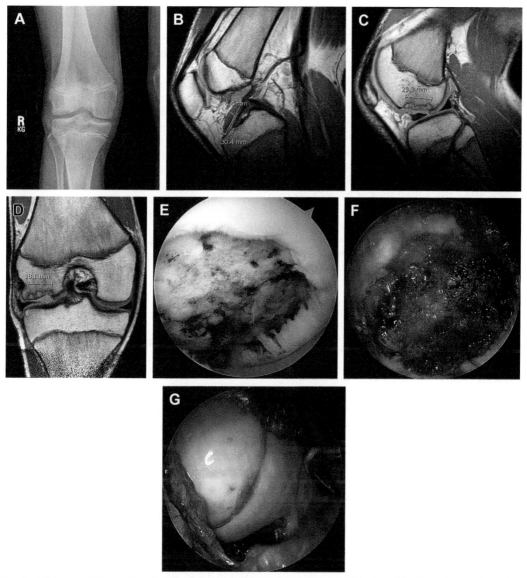

Fig. 1. A 14-year-old boy with a chronic unstable osteochondral defect (OCD) lesion of the lateral femoral condyle. (A) Preoperative anteroposterior radiograph showing the lesion. (B) Sagittal T1-weighted MRI through the notch showing unstable piece. (C) Sagittal T1-weighted MRI through the lateral femoral condyle showing lesion. (D) Coronal T1-weighted MRI showing the lesion with a cystic base. (E) Arthroscopic view of chronic OCD of the lateral femoral condyle. (F) Open view of chronic OCD after debridement and bone grafting from the ipsilateral proximal tibia. (G) Open view of OCD after fixation and bone grafting of the lesion.

limits its osteogenic and osteoinductive potential. Cancellous allografts are in the form of chips or croutons that can be used as bone-void fillers, and cortical allografts can provide rigid structural support; both require incorporation similar to their autogenous counterparts.[7]

More than 200,000 allografts are used in the United States each year, making them one of the most common orthobiologics used.[6,7] Advantages include the lack of donor site morbidity, decreased operative time, and decreased blood loss. They do, however, have higher costs than other alternatives and have the risk of viral and bacterial transmission. These rates are exceedingly low, but still should be mentioned.[2,7] Recent studies have shown a higher rate of rerupture in ACL reconstruction with the use of allografts in the pediatric population (MOON study [Multicenter Orthopedic Outcomes Network]).[10] Subsequently, allografts are used much more sparingly in children and are more common in adult patients.

AUTOLOGOUS BONE MARROW ASPIRATE

Autologous bone marrow is another source of orthobiologic material with osteogenic and osteoinductive properties with potential applications in sports medicine.[7,8] Bone marrow aspirate has a high concentration of MSCs that can be injected into the recipient site. It is easily obtainable from the iliac crest. One of the proposed theories for its effectiveness is that it also contains endothelial cell progenitor cells that can stimulate angiogenesis and restoration of blood flow at fracture sites. Bone marrow aspirate offers the advantages of being easy to obtain with much lower morbidity and fewer complications than other autologous grafts; however, it does not confer any structural support and can seep away from the intended target site because it is a liquid.[7] For this reason, it often is combined with other osteoconductive scaffolds such as DBX or ceramics.

BONE MORPHOGENIC PROTEIN

BMP was initially discovered almost 50 years ago. Since that time, more than 20 different proteins have been discovered. They are members of the transforming growth factor-β superfamily.[8] Their osteoinductive properties function as part of complex signaling pathways involved in osteoblastic differentiation and osteogenesis.[8,11] They have various functions, including osteoinductive activity, promoting cartilage formation, and promoting angiogenesis.[8] Two of the BMPs (BMP-2 and BMP-7) have proven to be effective in type I clinical studies of tibial fractures and nonunions and have been marketed for orthopedic use. Although their osteoinductive properties are inarguable, a number of complications have been reported, including renal or hepatic failure, heterotopic bone formation, wound complications, compartment syndrome, and carcinogenesis.[2] Furthermore, they are soluble proteins and have a tendency to dissipate from their graft sites, diluting their concentrations and potential effectiveness.[8] Despite this, the promising clinical outcomes of BMP have made it an intense research subject and major investment for industry.[8] The use of recombinant BMP in pediatric patients is currently off label, although the Food and Drug Administration has acknowledged that its use may be acceptable if the parents are fully informed.[2]

PLATELET-RICH PLASMA

PRP is an autologous suspension of platelets derived from a patient's whole blood with double centrifuge techniques.[7] It confers both osteogenic and osteoinductive properties. Once centrifuged, the platelets separate out into the layer above the erythrocytes.[12] The platelets are rich in key growth factors stored in the α-granule, including platelet-derived growth factor, transforming growth factor-β1, vascular endothelial growth factor, epidermal growth factor, fibroblast growth factor, and insulin-like growth factor-1. This extraction is then combined with calcium chloride to activate the platelets.[7] It can be injected into the host at that point to enhance stem cell recruitment, angiogenesis, and extracellular matrix production.[2] PRP has had some success in treating lateral epicondylitis and Achilles tendinopathy in adults. Its potential applications in sports medicine are still being studied extensively; however, no trials are specifically studying pediatric patients.

CERAMIC GRAFTS

Ceramic grafts are synthetic calcium salt–based substitutes that are alternatives to autologous and allogenic bone grafts. They are strictly osteoconductive, but can be combined with other orthobiologics. Ceramics are widely available at a relatively low cost and do not have the same risks with donor site morbidity and viral transmission risks as other types of graft.[7] Calcium sulfate, calcium phosphate, tricalcium phosphate, and coralline hydroxyapatite are all examples with slightly different resorption rates and characteristics. Several different forms are available, including powders, pellets, putty, blocks, and injectable forms. Ceramics are primarily marketed as bone void fillers and have been recommended for the treatment of unicameral bone cysts in the pediatric population.[2,8,13,14]

APPLICATIONS IN PEDIATRIC SPORTS MEDICINE

Orthobiologics have been widely used in sports medicine. ACL ruptures, cartilage damage, tendinopathies, and fractures are common musculoskeletal injuries affecting the young athletic population. Although much of the research involving orthobiologics and sports medicine has been done in adults, there are some studies that are pediatric specific or have transferrable results that can be applied to younger athletes.

LIGAMENT INJURIES

Ligamentous injuries and reconstructions in children and adolescents are increasing in numbers.

ACL reconstructions alone have increased at a rate of 924% from 1994 to 2006.[15] Year-round sports participation, the increasing number of athletes participating in sports, and more focus on a single sport are all theories of why this may be occurring.[16] Major ligamentous injuries in the pediatric population include the ACL, the medial patellofemoral ligament, and the ulnar collateral ligament (UCL).

Pediatric ACL injuries are typically seen in several forms: tibial spine avulsion fractures, partial ACL tears, and full-thickness ligament tears. The role for orthobiologics in these injuries is primarily for reconstruction of the ACL or augmentation of the repair, but some have advocated for their use in primary repair as well. Murray is currently working on a bridge enhanced ACL repair (BEAR [Bridge-Enhanced ACL Repair]) trial, where stitches and a bridging scaffold are used to stimulate healing in a torn ACL. These investigators have currently performed the surgery in 10 patients and preliminary results are promising, but still not definitive enough to recommend its routine use over reconstructive techniques.[17]

Graft choice has been studied extensively in the literature. Recent studies have shown that younger patients have an increased risk of ACL graft rupture and that the risk of rupture with allograft reconstruction is considerably higher than with autograft reconstruction.[18] The MOON cohort had a four times higher incidence of rerupture with allograft reconstruction compared with autograft reconstruction in 10- to 19-year-old patients (MOON).[10] The type of autograft used for ACL construction also varies. Choices include bone–patellar tendon–bone, quadriceps tendon, and hamstring autograft. Current recommendations from the academy show similar results in outcomes and strength of the grafts with bone–patellar tendon–bone and hamstring (American Academy of Orthopaedic Surgeons guidelines). Owing to concerns for placing bone across an open physis, soft tissue autografting has become the graft of choice in immature patients. In older adolescents, both hamstring and bone–patellar tendon–bone autografts can be used.[18,19] Additionally, the MOON looked at autograft size and the risk of revision and determined that larger soft tissue grafts (>8 mm) had less of a risk of rerupture.[20]

Other roles for orthobiologics in ACL reconstruction have focused on augmentation with osteoinductive substances such as PRP. One study by Vavken and colleagues[21] evaluated a biomaterial used in several large animal models of primary repair of partial and complete ACL transections. Researchers developed a collagen–platelet composite, which was placed into the wound site to enhance cellular proliferation and biosynthesis. Their findings showed promising functional outcomes when combined with primary repair.

Recent studies regarding the use of orthobiologics in ACL surgery in adults have reported mixed results. Figueroa and colleagues,[22] in a systematic review of PRP use in ACL surgery, found that although ACL graft maturity occurred more quickly with the use of PRP, there was no proof that the clinical outcomes of ACL surgery were enhanced by the use of PRP. Two other studies looked at graft incorporation via MRI signal after intraoperative use of PRP. Silva and colleagues[23] showed no difference at 3 months, whereas 6 months after hamstring autograft reconstruction Ventura and colleagues[24] noted differences in MRI signal density in grafts augmented with growth factors intraoperatively. Another cohort study by the MOON group evaluated augmentation of allograft ACL reconstructions with PRP at the end of the procedure[25] (Fig. 2). They found that, although effusions were decreased at 10 days in the PRP group, this difference disappeared by 8 weeks; there were no differences in patient-reported outcomes or number of additional surgeries at 2 years. This currently is an intense focus in research, but no definitive conclusions on the use of PRP in pediatric patients can be made at this time.

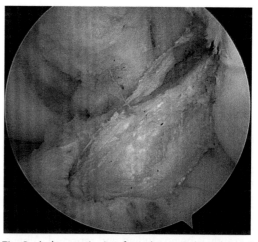

Fig. 2. Arthroscopic view from the anterolateral portal after reconstruction of the anterior cruciate ligament. The knee is lavaged and then platelet-rich plasma can be injected into the knee after closure and completion of the surgery.

The medial patellofemoral ligament is another common ligamentous reconstruction in children. Multiple reconstructive techniques have been described, but a common method involves reconstruction of the medial patellofemoral ligament with a hamstring graft. Rodriquez and colleagues[26] compared the clinical results of autograft with those of allograft reconstructions. They found comparable results and no significant differences between the groups with at least 12 months of follow-up. To our knowledge, no studies have looked at augmentation with orthobiologics in the pediatric population.

UCL injuries are increasingly prevalent in overhead throwing athletes. Surgical treatment options include UCL reconstruction with either tendon autograft or allograft. The use of orthobiologics in the treatment of partial UCL tears and to enhance recovery after reconstruction has become more frequent in adults. Two recent studies looked at using PRP injections to treat partial UCL tears in high-level throwing athletes. They found that the use of PRP produced outcomes much better than earlier reported outcomes of conservative treatment. Results indicated that PRP is an effective option to successfully treat partial UCL tears in the throwing athlete.[27,28] Hoffman and colleagues[29] used PRP and MSCs to augment surgical reconstruction of a UCL tear in professional baseball pitcher. Although follow-up has been limited, the patient has demonstrated excellent progress and returned to activity. Further research into the use of orthobiologics in the treatment of and enhancement of recovery from UCL injuries in the pediatric population is needed. Based on the current literature, the results are promising for the incorporation of orthobiologics in the treatment algorithm.

TENDON INJURIES

Tendinopathies and traumatic tendon injuries are common sports injuries in children and adolescents, but there is minimal clinical evidence currently available on the use of orthobiologics in pediatric tendon injuries. PRP and MSCs are increasingly becoming recognized in the treatment of adult musculoskeletal injuries, with recent reports of their being used to augment rotator cuff[30] and Achilles tendon repairs.[31] The use of orthobiologics in pediatric tendinosis, partial thickness tears, and interstitial tears currently is being studied and reported. Albano and colleagues[32] reported excellent results with the treatment of insertional patellar tendinosis with large complex interstitial tears in a 17-year-old basketball player with a combination

of PRP, bone marrow aspirate, and autologous fat graft from adipose-derived stem/stromal cells. They described using a therapeutic triad termed "autologous regenerative matrix." This autologous regenerative matrix injection is composed of:

1. PRP, which provides active cytokines and growth factors for wound healing and activation of progenitor cells;
2. Progenitor cells derived from lipoaspirants or, alternatively, bone marrow; and
3. A living bioscaffold provided by adipocytes and matrix derived from extracellular matrix and stromal vascular elements.

This autologous regenerative matrix is then transferred in the form of an injectable autologous graft. In another case study, Scollon-Grieve and colleagues[33] used ultrasound-guided injection of PRP into a nearly full-thickness patellar tendon tear in an 18-year-old lacrosse player in whom multiple other nonoperative treatments had failed and who had continued pain for nearly a year. At the 1-month follow-up the patient had 90% clinical improvement and a complete resolution of pain. Two months after the injection, he returned to full activity without pain or limitation.

CARTILAGE DEFECTS

Articular cartilage lesions pose a difficult challenge in adolescents, in whom the frequency of knee chondral injuries is high. Oepenn and colleagues,[34,35] in an MRI study, demonstrated that, after acute trauma, the most common injuries to the immature knee were chondral. Because adolescent cartilage has not yet calcified, forces are transmitted directly through the subchondral bone, resulting in an osteochondral fracture.[34,36,37] Large osteochondral fractures generally are treated with anatomic reduction and fixation. Repetitive microtrauma, osteochondritis dissecans, and chondromalacia patellae also are established causes of symptomatic articular lesions.[38–43] Not all lesions are symptomatic. With the aneural nature of articular cartilage, symptoms are believed to arise from the increased load on the subchondral bone. Asymptomatic lesions generally are treated nonoperatively because patients with an open distal femoral physis have a more favorable prognosis for healing. However, there is considerable evidence that symptomatic chondral defects should be treated.[34,44] Cartilage injuries to the adolescent knee are of particular concern because they may lead to premature osteoarthritis.[38] Articular cartilage has little capacity to repair itself or regenerate intrinsically.[45] Cartilage defects repair by forming scar tissue from the subchondral bone. This scar tissue is deficient in type II collagen and has "abnormal" proteoglycans (which have inferior biomechanical characteristics) and lower load-bearing capacity. Its formation often results in short-term recovery. Eventually, this surface can deteriorate and progress to produce chronic pain, poor function, and, in some cases, the early onset of osteoarthritis.[39,46]

Numerous treatments have been developed for the treatment of cartilage defects in the knee. Microfracture, osteochondral autograft, osteochondral allografts, and autologous chondrocyte implantation (ACI) are all well-described treatments with varying outcomes.[38,47–49] PRP is on the forefront of possible future treatment options used in articular cartilage injuries.

First described by Steadman and colleagues,[50] microfracture is a marrow-stimulating technique that involves the perforation of the subchondral bone. The aim is to release pluripotent stem cells from within the subchondral bone, along with growth factors and cytokines, to produce a clot rich in regenerative cells, an ideal environment for fibrocartilage repair.[39] Studies of pediatric patients have shown some good results. Knutson and colleagues,[51] in a randomized controlled study, suggested that microfracture produces results equivalent to those of ACI at 5 years. However, the technique produces fibrocartilage that does not possess the same properties as the lost hyaline cartilage and may not have the longevity of hyaline-type cartilage.[39,52] Best results have been shown in slim athletic patients with microfracture of the femoral condyle.[53] Some questions remain regarding its use in larger lesions, the repair material's long-term durability, and even the potential damage to the subchondral bone.[34,54,55]

Osteochondral autograft transplantation (OATS or mosaicplasty) involves the harvest of an osteochondral graft or grafts from a non–weight-bearing area of the knee and transplanting them into a defect. Two case series, including one observing more than 700 knees, have reported good results with osteochondral autograft transplantation.[39,56,57] Failures of this procedure have included donor site morbidity, inadequate filling of the defect, poor surface congruence, and failure of the mosaic plugs to integrate with the surrounding healthy cartilage.[39,44,58]

ACI aims to produce repair material resembling hyaline cartilage that can be used to treat articular cartilage defects. Three generations of ACI currently are used:

- First-generation, ACI with periosteal cover;
- Second-generation, ACI with type I/type III collagen-derived cover; and
- Third-generation, matrix-induced ACI.

DiBartola and colleagues,[38] in a systematic review of the clinical outcomes after ACI in adolescents' knees, found a 35.7% increase in clinical outcome scores from their preoperative level. Macmull and colleagues,[34] in a prospective study of 35 adolescents who underwent either ACI or matrix-induced ACI for symptomatic chondral and osteochondral lesions of the knee, found that pain and functional outcomes significantly improved despite the predominate repair material at 1 year being fibrocartilage. Two other studies also reported promising results with ACI treatment. Micheli and colleagues[59] performed a registry study of 37 adolescents undergoing ACI and demonstrated excellent and good results in 80% of patients. This study also found that patients with more than 4 years of follow-up reported greater improvements in their clinical outcomes scores than those with 2 to 4 years of follow-up. Mithofer and colleagues[34,60] assessed 20 adolescent athletes at a mean follow-up of 47 months after chondrocyte implantation for symptomatic chondral injuries: 96% of patients were able to return to high-impact sports and similarly 96% reported good or excellent results, and 60% reported return to sport at or above the preinjury level.[39,61] Interestingly, Mithofer and colleagues[34] reported that all patients returned to preinjury levels when the duration of symptoms was less than 12 months compared with only 33% who returned to preinjury level when the duration of symptoms was greater than 12 months. This demonstrates not only the potential for good outcomes in adolescents, but also the requirement for swift identification and treatment of the patient, particularly adolescent athletes. Teo and colleagues[38,61] reviewed 23 patients with a mean age of 16.8 years who had osteochondral defect of the patella treated with ACI or cultured bone marrow stem cell implantation. At a minimum follow-up of 2 years, there was significant improvement in KIDC scores, Lysholm scores, and Tegner scores. The current literature suggests that ACI provides clinical success across a number of different clinical outcomes measures when the technique is used in adolescent patients.

The use of osteochondral allografts includes harvesting articular cartilage grafts from cadavers and implanting them into chondral or osteochondral defects. Prospective cohort studies have shown good results with this technique.[34] As mentioned, the use of allografts carries some risks, including antigenicity, loss of mechanical strength, lack of osteoinductivity with sterilization techniques, and risk of transmitting viral and bacterial agents.[2,62]

PRP is another tool in the treatment of cartilage lesions. Recent reports in animal models suggest that the process of cartilage healing in vivo may be improved by local implantation of growth factors. These factors stimulate cell proliferation, migration, differentiation, and matrix synthesis and can affect chondrocyte metabolism and chondrogenesis and improve cartilage healing in vivo.[15,63–69] This would suggest that growth factors could be used to enhance cartilage repair. Sanchez and colleagues[12] described the use of PRP to augment Kirschner wire fixation of a large (>2 cm) articular cartilage avulsion fracture in an adolescent soccer player. They observed enhanced articular cartilage healing that led to an accelerated functional recovery. The patient returned to full competition and had complete healing of the cartilage lesion on MRI at 18 weeks. Although PRP represents a possible treatment option for the stimulation and acceleration of healing for cartilage lesions, at present there is little clinical evidence available to support its use. More evidence is necessary to determine the exact therapeutic value of PRP in regards to cartilage lesions.

FUTURE DIRECTION OF ORTHOBIOLOGICS IN PEDIATRIC SPORTS MEDICINE

Recent developments in orthobiologics have made it an intense focus of research within the field of orthopedic surgery. Practicing orthopedists require a working knowledge of autografts, allografts, bone graft substitutes, and other orthobiologics.[2] There is a paucity of research regarding their use in children. Indications in the adult population are being defined, but their applications can be expanded to children in certain situations.[2,4] The development and production of grafts, cell-based therapies, and bone graft substitutes have increased the options available to surgeons to promote more rapid healing. Expanding graft options, increasing graft incorporation, revascularizing tendon injuries, and cartilage repair and regeneration are all pressing problems in orthopedic surgery. Future direction of orthobiologics in pediatric sports medicine may include the ability to promote primary repair of injured ligaments, promote cartilage repair with less invasive techniques, shorten the time of return to sport, and decrease reinjury rates. Studies in the future will hopefully demonstrate clinical effectiveness and safety and will narrow indications to maximize their potential in the treatment of pediatric sports injuries.

REFERENCES

1. American Academy of Orthopaedic Surgeons. OrthoInfo. Available at: http://orthoinfo.aaos.org/topic.cfm?topic=A00525. Accessed December 1, 2016.
2. Gross RH. The use of bone grafts and bone graft substitutes in pediatric orthopaedics: an overview. J Pediatr Orthop 2012;32:100–5.
3. Markets and Markets. Orthobiologics. Available at: http://www.marketsandmarkets.com/Market-Reports/orthobiologics-market-162747970.html. Accessed December 1, 2016.
4. Richards BS, Oetgen ME, Johnston CE. The use of rhBMP-2 for the treatment of congenital pseudarthrosis of the tibia: a case series. J Bone Joint Surg Am 2010;92:177–85.
5. Myeroff C, Archdeacon M. Autogenous bone graft: donor sites and techniques. J Bone Joint Surg Am 2011;93(23):2227–36.
6. Khan SN, Cammisa FP Jr, Harvinder SS, et al. The biology of bone grafting. J Am Acad Orthop Surg 2005;13:77–86.
7. Roberts TT, Rosenbaum AJ. Bone grafts, bone substitutes and orthobiologics: the bridge between basic science and clinical advancements in fracture healing. Organogenesis 2012;8(4):114–24.
8. Finkemeier CG. Bone-grafting and bone-graft substitutes. J Bone Joint Surg Am 2002;84-A(3):454–64.
9. Flynn JM. Fracture repair and bone grafting. Rosemont (IL): American Academy of Orthopaedic Surgeons; 2011. p. 11–21.
10. Kaeding CC, Aros B, Pedroza A, et al. Allograft versus autograft anterior cruciate ligament reconstruction: predictors of failure from a MOON prospective longitudinal cohort. Sports Health 2011; 3:73–81.
11. Burwell RG. Studies in the transplantation of bone. VII. The composite homograft autograft of cancellous bone. An analysis of factors leading to osteogenesis in marrow transplants and marrow-containing bone grafts. J Bone Joint Surg Br 1964;46:110–40.
12. Sanchez M, Azofra J, Anitua E, et al. Plasma rich in growth factors to treat an articular cartilage avulsion: a case report. Med Sci Sports Exerc 2003; 35(10):1648–52.
13. Munting E, Wilmart JF, Wijne A, et al. Effect of sterilization of osteoinduction. Comparison of five

methods in demineralized rat bone. Acta Orthop Scand 1988;59:34–8.

14. Musculoskeletal Transplant Foundation. Edison, NJ. Available at: www.mtf.org.

15. Dekker TJ, Rush JK, Schmitz MR. What's new in pediatric and adolescent anterior cruciate ligament injuries. J Pediatr Orthop 2016. [Epub ahead of print].

16. Mall NA, Paletta GA. Pediatric ACL injuries: evaluation and management. Curr Rev Musculoskelet Med 2013;6(2):132–40.

17. Boston Children's Hospital, Boston, MA. BEAR trial. Available at: http://www.childrenshospital.org/centers-and-services/anterior-cruciate-ligament-program/bridge-enhanced-acl-repair-trial. Accessed February 16, 2017.

18. Fabricant PD, Jones KJ, Delos D, et al. Reconstruction of the anterior cruciate ligament in the skeletally immature athlete: a review of current concepts. J Bone Joint Surg Am 2013;95(5):e28.

19. Shea KG, Carey JL, Richmond J, et al. The American Academy of Orthopaedic Surgeons evidence-based guideline on management of anterior cruciate ligament injuries. J Bone Joint Surg Am 2015;97:672–4.

20. Mariscalco MW, Flanigan DC, Mitchell J, et al. The influence of hamstring autograft size on patient reported outcomes and risk of revision following anterior cruciate ligament reconstruction: a MOON cohort study. Arthroscopy 2013;29(12):1948–53.

21. Vavken P, Murray MM. The potential for primary repair of the ACL. Sports Med Arthrosc 2011;19(1):44–9.

22. Figueroa D, Figueroa F, Calvo R, et al. Platelet-rich plasma use in anterior cruciate ligament surgery: systematic review of the literature. Arthroscopy 2015;31(5):981–8.

23. Silva A, Sampaio R. Anatomic ACL reconstruction: does platelet-rich plasma accelerate tendon healing? Knee Surg Sports Traumatol Arthrosc 2009;17:676–82.

24. Ventura A, Terzaghi C, Borgo E, et al. Use of growth factors in ACL surgery: preliminary study. J Orthop Trauma 2005;6:76–9.

25. Magnussen RA, Flanigan DC, Pedroza AD, et al. Platelet rich plasma use in allograft ACL reconstructions: two-year clinical results of a MOON cohort study. Knee 2013;20(4):277–80.

26. Calvo RR, Figueroa PD, Anastasiadis LZ, et al. Reconstruction of the medial patellofemoral ligament: evaluation of the clinical results of autografts versus allografts. Rev Esp Cir Ortop Traumatol 2015;59(5):348–53.

27. Dines JS, Williams PN, ElAttrache N, et al. Platelet-rich plasma can be used to successfully treat elbow ulnar collateral ligament insufficiency in high-level throwers. Am J Orthop 2016;45(5):296–300.

28. Podesta L, Crow SA, Volkmer D, et al. Treatment of partial ulnar collateral ligament tears in the elbow with platelet-rich plasma. Am J Sports Med 2013;41(7):1689–94.

29. Hoffman JK, Protzman NM, Malhotra AD. Biologic augmentation of the ulnar collateral ligament in the elbow of a professional baseball pitcher. Case Rep Orthop 2015;2015:130157.

30. Sanchez M, Anitua E, Azofra J, et al. Comparison of surgically repaired Achilles tendon tears using platelet-rich fibrin matrices. Am J Sports Med 2007;35:245–51.

31. Randelli PS, Arrigoni P, Cabitza P, et al. Autologous platelet rich plasma for arthroscopic rotator cuff repair: a pilot study. Disabil Rehabil 2008;30:1584–9.

32. Albano JJ, Alexander RW. Autologous fat grafting as a mesenchymal stem cell source and living bioscaffold in a patellar tendon tear. Clin J Sport Med 2011;21(4):359–61.

33. Scollon-Grieve KL, Malanga GA. Platelet-rich plasma injection for partial patellar tendon tear in a high school athlete: a case presentation. PM R 2011;3:391–5.

34. Macmull S, Parratt M, Bentley G, et al. Autologous chondrocyte implantation in the adolescent knee. Am J Sports Med 2011;39(8):1723–30.

35. Oepenn RS, Connolly SA, Bencardino JT, et al. Acute injury of the articular cartilage and subchondral bone: a common but unrecognized lesion in the immature knee. AJR Am J Roentgenol 2004;182:111–7.

36. Landells JW. The reactions of injured human articular cartilage. J Bone Joint Surg Br 1957;39:548–62.

37. Rosenberg NJ. Osteochondral fractures of the lateral femoral condyle. J Bone Joint Surg Am 1964;46:1013–26.

38. DiBartola AC, Wright BM, Magnussen RA, et al. Clinical outcomes after autologous chondrocyte implantation in adolescent's knees: a systematic review. Arthroscopy 2016;32(9):1905–16.

39. Macmull S, Skinner JA, Bentley G, et al. Treating articular cartilage injuries of the knee in young people. BMJ 2010;340:c998.

40. Bollen S. Epidemiology of knee injuries: diagnosis and triage. Br J Sports Med 2000;34:227–8.

41. Noyes FR, Bassett RW, Grood ES, et al. Arthroscopy in acute traumatic hemarthrosis of the knee. incidence of anterior cruciate tears and other injuries. J Bone Joint Surg Am 1980;62:687–95, 757.

42. Peers SC, Maerz T, Baker EA, et al. T1 rho magnetic resonance imaging for detection of early cartilage changes in knees of asymptomatic collegiate female impact and nonimpact athletes. Clin J Sport Med 2014;24:218–25.

43. Krishnan SP, Skinner JA, Carrington RW, et al. Collagen-covered autologous chondrocyte implantation for osteochondritis dissecans of the knee: two to seven-year results. J Bone Joint Surg Br 2006;88:203–5.

44. Smith GD, Knutson G, Richardson JB. A clinical review of cartilage repair techniques. J Bone Joint Surg Br 2005;87:445–9.

45. Mankin HJ. The response of articular cartilage to mechanical injury. J Bone Joint Am 1982;64:460–6.

46. Buckwalter JA. Articular cartilage injuries. Clin Orthop Relat Res 2002;402:21–37.

47. Niemeyer P, Porichis S, Steinwachs M, et al. Long-term outcomes after first generation autologous chondrocyte implantation for cartilage defects of the knee. Am J Sports Med 2014;42:150–7.

48. Steadman JR, Briggs KK, Matheny LM, et al. Outcomes following microfracture of full-thickness articular cartilage lesions of the knee in adolescent patients. J Knee Surg 2015;28:145–50.

49. Shaha JS, Cook JB, Rowles DJ, et al. Return to an athletic lifestyle after osteochondral allograft transplantation of the knee. Am J Sports Med 2013;41: 2083–9.

50. Steadman JR, Rodkey WG, Singleton SB, et al. Microfracture: surgical technique for full thickness chondral defects: technique and clinical results. Oper Tech Orthop 1997;7:300–4.

51. Knutson G, Drogset JO, Engebretsen L, et al. A randomized trial comparing autologous chondrocyte implantation with microfracture: findings at five years. J Bone Joint Surg Am 2007;89(10): 2105–12.

52. Hunziker EB. Articular cartilage repair: basic science and clinical progress: a review of the current status and prospects. Osteoarthritis Cartilage 2002;10:432–6.

53. Kreuz PC, Steinwachs MR, Erggelet C, et al. Results after microfracture of full-thickness chondral defects in different compartments in the knee. Osteoarthritis Cartilage 2006;14(11):1119–25.

54. Minas T, Gomoll AH, Rosenberger R, et al. Increased failure rate of autologous chondrocyte implantation after previous treatment with marrow stimulation techniques. Am J Sports Med 2009;37: 902–8.

55. Minas T, Nehrer S. Current concepts in the treatment of articular cartilage defects. Orthopedics 1997;20:525–38.

56. Hangody L, Fules P. Autologous osteochondral mosaicplasty for the treatment of full-thickness defects of weight-bearing joints: ten years of experimental and clinical experience. J Bone Joint Surg Am 2003;85(Suppl 2):25–32.

57. Chow JC, Hantes ME, Houle JB, et al. Arthroscopic autogenous osteochondral transplantation for treating knee cartilage defects: a 2-5 year follow-up study. Arthroscopy 2004;20:681–90.

58. Bentley G, Biant LC, Carrington RW, et al. A prospective, randomized comparison of autologous chondrocyte implantation versus mosaicplasty for osteochondral defects in the knee. J Bone Joint Surg Br 2003;85-B:223–30.

59. Micheli LJ, Moseley JB, Anderson AF, et al. Articular cartilage defects of the distal femur in children and adolescents: treatment with autologous chondrocyte implantation. J Pediatr Orthop 2006;26:455–60.

60. Mithofer K, Minas T, Peterson L, et al. Functional outcome of knee articular cartilage repair in adolescent athletes. Am J Sports Med 2005;33:1147–53.

61. Teo BJ, Buhary K, Tai BC, et al. Cell-based therapy improves function in adolescents and young adults with patellar osteochondritis dissecans. Clin Orthop Relat Res 2013;471:1152–8.

62. Beebe KS, Benevenia J, Tuy BT, et al. Effects of a new allograft processing procedure on graft healing in a canine model. Clin Orthop Relat Res 2009;467:273–80.

63. Buckwalter JA, Mankin HJ. Articular cartilage: degeneration and osteoarthritis, repair, regeneration, and transplantation. Instr Course Lect 2008; 47:487–504.

64. Frenkel SR, Saadeh PB, Mehrara BJ, et al. Transforming growth factor beta superfamily members: role in cartilage modeling. Plast Reconstr Surg 2000;105:980–90.

65. Hiraki Y, Shukunami C, Iyama K, et al. Differentiation of chondrogenic precursor cells during the regeneration of articular cartilage. Osteoarthritis Cartilage 2001;9:S102–8.

66. Lee KH, Song SU, Hwang TS, et al. Regeneration of hyaline cartilage by cell-mediating gene therapy using transforming growth factor beta 1-producing fibroblasts. Hum Gene Ther 2001;12:1805–13.

67. Martinek V, Fu FH, Huard J. Gene therapy and tissue engineering in sports medicine. Phys Sportsmed 2000;28:34–51.

68. Martinek V, Fu FH, Lee CW, et al. Treatment of osteochondral injuries: genetic engineering. Clin Sports Med 2001;20:403–16.

69. Van Der Berg WB, Van der Kraan PM, Scharstuhl A, et al. Growth factors and cartilage repair. Clin Orthop 2001;391:S224–50.

Upper Extremity

Biologic Approaches to Problems of the Hand and Wrist

Murphy M. Steiner, MD*, James H. Calandruccio, MD

KEYWORDS

- Orthobiologics • Hand • Wrist • PRP • BMP • Kienböck disease

KEY POINTS

- Orthobiologics are not used as frequently in the hand and wrist as in other sites.
- The most frequently reported is the use of bone morphogenetic protein for the treatment of Kienböck disease.
- Animal studies have described improved tendon healing with the use of platelet-rich plasma (PRP), but no clinical studies have confirmed these results.
- PRP has been reported to produce improvements in the outcomes of distal radial fractures and osteoarthritis of the trapeziometacarpal in small numbers of patients.
- The use of orthobiologics in the hand and wrist has just begun to be explored, and the applications are promising, but clinical trials are necessary to establish efficacy and safety.

Although not as frequently used as in other sites, biologic solutions have been sought for a variety of orthopedic conditions in the hand and wrist, including Kienböck disease; scaphoid, distal radial, ulnar, and phalangeal fractures and nonunions; osteochondral lesions of the capitate; and thumb arthritis.

BONE MORPHOGENETIC PROTEIN

Kienböck Disease

Kienböck disease, first described in 1910 as "lunatomalacia," is osteonecrosis of the carpal lunate postulated to be caused by trauma with disruption of the blood supply to the lunate; however, no single cause has been identified and the exact mechanism of vascular impairment remains unclear. Other factors that may be involved in Kienböck disease include variations in skeletal development causing an irregular size or shape of the ulna, radius, or lunate, and medical conditions that affect blood supply, such as lupus, sickle cell anemia, and cerebral palsy. Progressive deterioration of the lunate causes pain and limits motion. When symptoms are unrelieved by nonoperative methods, operative treatment is indicated and may involve revascularization, joint leveling, proximal row carpectomy, or wrist fusion. Revascularization procedures are most commonly chosen for young, active patients for whom loss of wrist motion would be incapacitating and most often includes curettage of avascular bone from the lunate and placement of a vascularized bone graft. Bone morphogenetic proteins (BMP), both human (hBMP) and recombinant (rhBMP) forms, have been shown to induce bony healing in animal and human studies. BMPs have been successfully used in the treatment of open tibial fractures,[1] spinal fusions,[2] and nonunions.[3–5] Jones and colleagues[6] described improved range of motion, complete resolution of pain, and no further lunate collapse at 6 years after the use of hBMP with vascular pedicle implantation in a patient with stage IIIA Kienböck

---

The authors have nothing to disclose.
Department of Orthopaedic Surgery and Biomedical Engineering, University of Tennessee-Campbell Clinic, 1211 Union Avenue, Suite 510, Memphis, TN 38104, USA
* Corresponding author.
E-mail address: murphysteiner@gmail.com

disease. Rajfer and colleagues[7] reported arthroscopic curettage and grafting with a mixture of autologous radial cancellous bone marrow graft and BMP-2 in 2 patients (3 wrists) with stage III Kienböck disease, all of which had favorable results. They suggested this technique of arthroscopic curettage, bone grafting, and adjunctive BMP as a minimally invasive alternative to radial osteotomy in patients who do not have pathologic ulnar-negative variance.

Fractures/Nonunions

Two studies of the use of BMP in the treatment of scaphoid nonunions reached opposing conclusions (Table 1). In one, Bilic and colleagues[8] randomly assigned 17 patients with scaphoid nonunions to treatment with autologous iliac graft, autologous iliac graft plus osteogenic protein (OP-1; Osigraft), or allogeneic iliac graft plus OP-1. At 2-year follow-up, they found that OP-1 improved the performance of both autologous and allogeneic bone implants. Computed tomography scanning and scintigraphy showed that sclerotic bone was replaced by well-vascularized bone in patients treated with OP-1. Radiographic healing time was reduced to 4 weeks in those with autologous grafts plus OP-1 compared with the groups with autologous iliac grafts alone. Patients with allogeneic grafts plus OP-1 had radiographic healing at 8 weeks, which was comparable to the healing time in patients with autologous graft alone. These investigators suggested that, because the addition of OP-1 to allogeneic bone produced clinical outcomes equal to those obtained with autologous graft, harvesting of autologous bone from the iliac crest might be avoided.

Contrary to these results, Rice and Lubahn[9] found that the addition of rhBMP-2 to surgical repair of 27 hand and wrist nonunions (phalanx, carpus, distal radius and ulna) resulted in radiographic union rates consistent with previously published rates and did not produce superior rates of union in their patients. Of 6 patients with scaphoid nonunions treated with rhBMP-2 by Brannan and colleagues,[10] 2 required scaphoid excision and midcarpal arthrodesis and 4 developed notable heterotopic ossification,

Table 1 Researched applications of BMP in hand surgery			
Authors	**Clinical Application**	**Purpose**	**Outcome**
Jones et al,[6] 2008	Kienböck disease	Report a case of BMP used in combination with vascularized pedicle bone graft	Imaging demonstrated successful revascularization. Patient had resolution of pain and improved range of motion.
Rajfer et al,[7] 2013	Kienböck disease	Describe an arthroscopic technique to treat using autograft with BMP-2	Authors performed this technique in 2 patients (3 wrists) for stage IIIA and IIIB Kienböck disease with favorable results.
Bilic et al,[8] 2006	Scaphoid nonunion	Randomized trial comparing iliac bone graft with and without OP-1 (BMP-7)	OP-1 improved healing time of autograft. Healing time was similar for autograft and allograft with OP-1.
Rice & Lubahn,[9] 2013	Nonunions of hand/wrist	Compare radiographic union rates of historical controls with BMP in addition to surgical repair	The use of BMP-2 did not increase the radiographic union rate when used with surgical repair compared with surgery alone.
Brannan et al,[10] 2016	Revision scaphoid nonunion	To identify complications resulting from BMP use in a revision scaphoid nonunion ORIF	Use of BMP-2 was associated with higher complication rates than previously described. They include heterotopic ossification, persistent nonunion, and loss of ROM.

Abbreviations: BMP, bone morphogenetic protein; OP, osteogenic protein; ORIF, open reduction internal fixation; ROM, range of motion.

prompting these investigators to advise consideration of the potential complications, especially heterotopic ossification, when using rhBMP-2.

PLATELET-RICH PLASMA

Platelet-rich plasma (PRP) is another biologic preparation believed to positively influence the body's natural healing process. Its effectiveness is based on a high level of growth factors, including platelet-derived growth factor, transforming growth factor-b (TGF-b), fibroblastic growth factor (FGF), vascular endothelial growth factor (VEGF), insulinlike growth factor-1 (IGF-1), and epidermal growth factor. PRP has been widely used in a variety of orthopedic applications, including fractures and nonunions; spine fusions; and cartilage, tendon, and ligament injuries.[11,12] Its use in the upper extremity has been primarily limited to the treatment of tendinopathies at the elbow (lateral epicondylitis, distal biceps tendinopathy) and to rotator cuff repairs.[13,14]

Because of concerns that PRP may increase performance-enhancing growth factors, the World Anti-Doping Agency (WADA) banned intramuscular PRP injections in competitive athletes in 2010. This ban was lifted in 2011 because there was limited evidence of a systemic ergogenic effect, but the growth factors within PRP remain prohibited. Wasterlain and colleagues[15] found a statistically significant increase in circulating concentrations of VEGF, IGF-1, and basic FGF after a single injection of leukocyte-rich PRP, all of which are currently banned, as of the 2017 WADA Prohibited List, in competitive athletes.

Tendons

Animal studies of the use PRP to improve tendon healing in other upper extremity sites have had varying outcomes (Table 2).[16–19] Sato and colleagues,[19] in a rabbit model, demonstrated a statistically significant increase in flexor tendon tensile strength with the addition of PRP-impregnated fibrin matrix to tendon repair. In contrast, Kollitz and colleagues[18] found that PRP did not improve ultimate tensile strength of zone II flexor tendon repairs in a rabbit model; in fact, PRP-treated tendons tended to have decreased tensile strength compared with controls. They also did not observe any significant effects of PRP on range of motion or tendon excursion. Calandruccio and colleagues[17] compared the effects of saline, steroid, autologous blood, and PRP on the strength and structure of the Achilles tendon in a rat tendinopathy model and found no significant difference in tendon strength among treatment groups, although the autologous blood injection group had the greatest load-to-failure value and the PRP and saline groups had significantly lower load-to-failure values.[17] Autologous blood injection appeared to improve tendon strength and promote a more substantial histologic response, whereas PRP and steroid treatment seemed to weaken tendons while not producing a significant histologic improvement.

The differences in outcomes of PRP treatment of tendons may be due in large part to the differences in PRP preparation, particularly the concentration of leukocytes. Zhang and colleagues,[20] in a laboratory study, showed that leukocyte-rich PRP (L-PRP) actually had a detrimental effect on tendon stem cells. Although tendon stem cells cultured in pure PRP without leukocytes produced more collagen and formed tendonlike tissue, tendon stem cells grown in L-PRP differentiated into nontenocytes and produced more inflammatory factors, such as membrane-associated prostaglandin synthase and interleukin (IL)-1ß. L-PRP also was associated with increased apoptosis. These effects were confirmed in a study of rabbit patellar tendons in which L-PRP induced catabolic and inflammatory effects on tendon cells.[21]

Fractures

A recent randomized trial by Namazi and Mehbudi[22] of 30 distal radial fractures, all treated with closed reduction and percutaneous pinning, compared outcomes of 15 patients who received PRP injections into the radiocarpal joint with those of 15 patients who did not receive PRP injections. They found significant improvements in pain and activity scores in the PRP group but no statistically significant difference in wrist motion.

Osteoarthritis

Based on the reported success of PRP injections for osteoarthritis (OA) of the knee, Loibl and colleagues[23] used leukocyte-reduced PRP for treatment of OA of the trapeziometacarpal joint in 10 patients. At 6-month follow-up, 2 patients were very satisfied with their results, 5 were satisfied, and 3 were neither satisfied nor dissatisfied. Patients with mild-to-moderate OA had decreased pain and improvements in the Disabilities of the Arm, Shoulder and Hand (DASH) and Mayo Wrist scores that persisted at the 6-month follow-up; patients with more severe OA did not experience lasting benefit.

Table 2
Researched applications of PRP in hand surgery

Authors	Site of Application	Model	Purpose	Outcome
Sato et al,[19] 2012	Flexors tendon	Rabbit	Evaluate effect of PRP fibrin matrix on tendon repair	PRP fibrin matrix significantly increased tensile strength of flexor tendon repair.
Kollitz et al,[18] 2014	Flexor tendon	Rabbit	Evaluate effect of PRP on strength of zone II repairs	PRP decreased tensile strength repair compared with controls.
Calandruccio et al,[17] 2015	Achilles tendon	Rat	Compare effects of saline, steroid, AB, and PRP on Achilles tendon	Saline and PRP groups had statistically lower loads-to-failure. The AB group showed a trend toward higher load-to-failure.
Zhang et al,[20] 2016	Tendon stem cells	In vitro	Compare effects of leukocyte-rich and pure PRP on tendon stem cells	Stem cells with pure PRP produced more tendonlike tissue, fewer inflammatory factors, and less apoptosis.
Zhou et al,[21] 2015	Patellar tendon	Rabbit	Determine the effects of leukocyte-rich and pure PRP on tendon stem cells	Leukocyte-rich PRP had catabolic and inflammatory effects, whereas pure PRP induced anabolic changes. Both types induced tenocyte differentiation.
Namazi & Mehbudi,[22] 2016	Radiocarpal joint	In vivo	Evaluate effect of wrist PRP injection in the setting of intra-articular distal radius fracture	Intra-articular PRP injection was associated with improved pain and activity scores with 3-month follow-up. Wrist motion was not different.
Loibl et al,[23] 2016	Trapeziometacarpal joint	In vivo	Investigate pain relief with PRP for basal joint osteoarthritis	Patients with mild-to-moderate OA had improved pain, DASH, and Mayo scores up to 6 mo. PRP was not effective in severe OA.

Abbreviations: AB, autologous blood; DASH, Disabilities of the Arm, Shoulder, and Hand; OA, osteoarthritis; PRP, platelet-rich plasma.

de Quervain Tenosynovitis

Because of favorable results reported with the use of PRP in other tendinopathies (eg, Achilles, elbow, patellar, rotator cuff), Peck and Ely[24] used ultrasound-guided percutaneous needle tenotomy and PRP injection for the treatment of de Quervain tenosynovitis in one patient, a 74-year-old woman, in whom 3 months of conservative treatment with activity modifications, bracing, occupational therapy, and ultrasound-guided corticosteroid injections failed to relieve pain. At 6 months after the procedure, she had a 63% reduction in pain according to her Visual Analog Scale score. No complications were noted during the procedure or in the following 6 months.

STEM CELLS

Stem cells by definition are undifferentiated cells that have 4 main characteristics:

- Mobilization during angiogenesis
- Differentiation into specialized cell types
- Proliferation and regeneration
- Release of immune regulators and growth factors

Both bone marrow–derived mesenchymal stem cells (MSCs) and adipose-derived MSCs are multipotent stem cells that originate from mesenchymal tissues, such as bone marrow, tendons, adipose tissue, periosteum, and muscle tissue. The source tissue used to isolate MSCs can affect differentiation capabilities, colony size, and growth rate.

Most studies of the use of MSCs in structures analogous to the human hand and wrist have been done in animal models.[25,26] Evaluation of 141 race horses with superficial digital flexor tendinopathy treated with MSCs found a reinjury rate of 27.4%, a rate similar to historical controls.[27] Another study, however, of collagen fibril size after treatment of superficial digital flexor tendon injuries in horses found no measurable effect from the use of MSCs.[28] Treatment of Kienböck disease in a rabbit model has been described in several studies, with abundant neovascularization and maintenance of carpal height.[29–32]

Clinical trials have involved primarily Achilles and patellar tendon injuries, rotator cuff, and tennis elbow. Granel and colleagues[33] and Guillaume-Jugnot and colleagues[34] described the use of autologous adipose-derived stromal vascular fraction in patients with hand disabilities due to systemic sclerosis and found significant improvements in hand disability and pain,

Raynaud phenomenon, finger swelling, and quality of life. Tissue repair cells from bone marrow were used by Comerota and colleagues[35] to treat a patient with bilateral hand gangrene; intramuscular injections resulted in increased arterial perfusion, elimination of ischemic rest pain, and healing of all previously gangrenous digital amputation sites.

Although many studies over the past decade have described the safe use of MSCs to treat orthopedic conditions, there is still concern about the possibility of malignant transformation. Centeno and colleagues[36] reported the results of 3 treatment registry studies that followed complications in 227 (2010) and 339 (2011)[37] orthopedic patients treated with culture-expanded MSCs; no neoplastic complications were noted at any stem-cell implantation site. More recently, they reviewed a registry database that included 2372 patients followed for up to 9 years.[38] Among these patients, only 7 (0.3%) had reported neoplasms, a lower rate than in the general population.

SUMMARY

There is conflicting evidence regarding the use of orthobiologics in hand surgery. Although there are animal models with encouraging results, clinical success has not been as well documented as in some other areas of orthopedics. Further research is required to determine the clinical benefit of the various orthobiologics in hand surgery.

REFERENCES

1. Govender S, Csimma C, Genant HK, et al. Recombinant human bone morphogenetic protein-2 for treatment of open tibial fractures: a prospective, controlled, randomized study of four hundred and fifty patients. J Bone Joint Surg Am 2002;84: 2123–34.

2. Boden SD, Kang J, Sandhu H, et al. Use of recombinant human bone morphogenetic protein-2 to achieve posterolateral lumbar spine fusion in humans: a prospective, randomized clinical pilot trial: 2002 Volvo award in clinical studies. Spine (Phila Pa 1976) 2000;27:2662–73.

3. Friedlaender GE, Perry CR, Cole JD, et al. Osteogenic protein-1 (bone morphogenetic protein-7) in the treatment of tibial nonunions. J Bone Joint Surg Am 2001;83-A(Suppl 1(Pt 2)):S151–8.

4. Johnson EE, Urist MR. Human bone morphogenetic protein allografting for reconstruction of femoral nonunion. Clin Orthop Relat Res 2000;(371):61–74.

5. Jones NF, Brown EE, Mostofi A, et al. Healing of a scaphoid nonunion using bone morphogenetic protein. J Hand Surg Am 2005;30:528–33.

6. Jones NF, Brown EE, Vögelin E, et al. Bone morphogenetic protein as an adjuvant in the treatment of Kienböck's disease by vascular pedicle implantation. J Hand Surg Eur Vol 2008;33:317–21.

7. Rajfer RA, Danoff JR, Metzl JA, et al. A novel arthroscopic technique utilizing bone morphogenetic protein in the treatment of Kienböck disease. Tech Hand Up Exterm Surg 2013;17:2–6.

8. Bilic R, Simic P, Jelic H, et al. Osteogenic protein-1 (BMP-7) accelerates healing of scaphoid non-union with proximal pole sclerosis. Int Orthop 2006;30:128–34.

9. Rice I, Lubahn JD. Use of bone morphogenetic protein-2 (rh-BMP-2) in treatment of wrist and hand nonunion with comparison to historical control groups. J Surg Orthop Adv 2013;22:256–62.

10. Brannan PS, Gaston RG, Loeffler BJ, et al. Complications with the use of BMP-2 in scaphoid nonunion surgery. J Hand Surg Am 2016;41:602–8.

11. Baksh N, Hannon CP, Murawski CD, et al. Platelet-rich plasma in tendon models: a systematic review of basic science literature. Arthroscopy 2013;29:596–607.

12. Hsu WK, Mishra A, Rodeo SR, et al. Platelet-rich plasma in orthopaedic applications: evidence-based recommendations for treatment. J Am Acad Orthop Surg 2013;21:739–48.

13. Mishra A, Randelli P, Barr C, et al. Platelet-rich plasma and the upper extremity. Hand Clin 2012;28:481–91.

14. Randelli P, Arrigoni P, Ragone V, et al. Platelet-rich plasma in arthroscopic rotator cuff repair: a prospective RCT study, 2-year follow-up. J Shoulder Elbow Surg 2011;20:518–28.

15. Wasterlain AS, Braun HJ, Harris AH, et al. The systemic effects of platelet-rich plasma injection. Am J Sports Med 2013;41:186–93.

16. Bosch G, van Schie HT, de Groot MW, et al. Effects of platelet-rich plasma on the quality of repair of mechanically induced core lesions in equine superficial digital flexor tendons: a placebo-controlled experimental study. J Orthop Res 2010;28:211–7.

17. Calandruccio JH, Cannon TA, Wodowski AJ, et al. A mechanical and histologic comparative study of the effect of saline steroid, autologous blood, and platelet-rich plasma on collagenase-induced Achilles tendinopathy in a rat model. Curr Orthop Prac 2015;26:E7–12.

18. Kollitz KM, Parsons EM, Weaver MS, et al. Platelet-rich plasma for zone II flexor tendon repair. Hand (N Y) 2014;9:217–24.

19. Sato D, Takahara M, Narita A, et al. Effect of platelet-rich plasma with fibrin matrix on healing of intrasynovial flexor tendons. J Hand Surg Am 2012;37:1356–63.

20. Zhang L, Chen S, Chang P, et al. Harmful effects of leukocyte-rich platelet-rich plasma on rabbit tendon stem cells in vitro. Am J Sports Med 2016;44:1941–51.

21. Zhou Y, Zhang J, Wu H, et al. The differential effects of leukocyte-containing and pure platelet-rich plasma (PRP) on tendon stem/progenitor cells–implications of PRP application for the clinical treatment of tendon injuries. Stem Cell Res Ther 2015;6:173.

22. Namazi H, Mehbudi A. Investigating the effect of intra-articular PRP injection on pain and function improvement in patients with distal radius fracture. Orthop Traumatol Surg Res 2016;102:47–52.

23. Loibl M, Lang S, Dendel LM, et al. Leukocyte-reduced platelet-rich plasma treatment of basal thumb arthritis: a pilot study. Biomed Res Int 2016;2016:9262909.

24. Peck E, Ely E. Successful treatment of de Quervain tenosynovitis with ultrasound-guided percutaneous needle tenotomy and platelet-rich plasma injection: a case presentation. PM R 2013;5:438–41.

25. Chong AK, He M. Stem cells and biological approaches to treatment of wrist problems. J Wrist Surg 2013;2:315–8.

26. He M, Gan AW, Lim AY, et al. Bone marrow derived mesenchymal stem cell augmentation of rabbit flexor tendon healing. Hand Surg 2015;20:421–9.

27. Godwin EE, Young NJ, Dudhia J, et al. Implantation of bone marrow-derived mesenchymal stem cells demonstrates improved outcome in horses with overstrain injury of the superficial digital flexor tendon. Equine Vet J 2012;44:25–32.

28. Caniglia CJ, Schramme MC, Smith RK. The effect of intralesional injection of bone marrow derived mesenchymal stem cells and bone marrow supernatant on collagen fibril size in a surgical model of equine superficial digital flexor tendonitis. Equine Vet J 2012;44:587–93.

29. Berner A, Pfaller C, Dienstknecht T, et al. Arthroplasty of the lunate using bone marrow mesenchymal stromal cells. Int Orthop 2011;35:379–87.

30. Huang JI, Durbhakula MM, Angele P, et al. Lunate arthroplasty with autologous mesenchymal stem cells in a rabbit model. J Bone Joint Surg Am 2006;88:744–52.

31. Ogawa T, Ishii T, Mishima H, et al. Effectiveness of bone marrow transplantation for revitalizing a severely necrotic small bone: experimental rabbit model. J Orthop Sci 2010;15:381–8.

32. Shigematsu K, Hattori K, Kobata Y, et al. Treatment of Kienböck's disease with cultured stem cell-seeded hybrid tendon roll interposition arthroplasty: experimental study. J Orthop Sci 2006;11:198–203.

33. Granel B, Daumas A, Jouve E, et al. Safety, tolerability and potential efficacy of injection of autologous adipose-derived stromal vascular fraction in the fingers of patients with systemic sclerosis: an open-label phase I trial. Ann Rheum Dis 2015;74:2175–82.

34. Guillaume-Jugnot P, Daumas A, Magalon J, et al. Autologous adipose-derived stromal vascular fraction in patients with systemic sclerosis: 12-month follow-up. Rheumatology (Oxford) 2016;55:301–6.

35. Comerota A, Link A, Douville J, et al. Upper extremity ischemia treated with tissue repair cells from adult bone marrow. J Vasc Surg 2010;52:723–9.

36. Centeno CJ, Schultz JR, Cheever M, et al. Safety and complications reporting update on the re-implantation of culture-expanded mesenchymal stem cells using autologous platelet lysate technique. Curr Stem Cell Res Ther 2010;5:81–93.

37. Centeno CJ, Schultz JR, Cheever M, et al. Safety and complications reporting update on the re-implantation of culture-expanded mesenchymal stem cells using autologous platelet lysate technique. Curr Stem Cell Res 2011;6:368–78.

38. Centeno CJ, Al-Satyegh H, Freeman MD, et al. A multi-center analysis of adverse events among two thousand, three hundred and seventy two adult patients undergoing adult autologous stem cell therapy for orthopaedic conditions. Int Orthop 2016;40:1755–65.

Autologous Blood and Platelet-Rich Plasma Injections for Treatment of Lateral Epicondylitis

James H. Calandruccio, MD, Murphy M. Steiner, MD*

KEYWORDS

- Lateral epicondylitis • Tennis elbow • Autologous blood injection • Platelet-rich plasma
- Outcomes

KEY POINTS

- Lateral epicondylitis (tennis elbow) is a frequent cause of elbow pain; most patients (80%–90%) are successfully treated with standard nonoperative methods (rest, nonsteroidal anti-inflammatory drugs, bracing, and physical therapy).
- Autologous blood injections (ABI) and platelet-rich plasma (PRP) injections are the two most frequently used orthobiologic techniques in the treatment of lateral epicondylitis (tennis elbow).
- Studies of the effectiveness of ABI and PRP report varying outcomes, some citing significant clinical relief and others reporting no beneficial effect.
- More research is needed to determine how to best use orthobiologics in the treatment of lateral epicondylitis.

Lateral epicondylitis (tennis elbow) is a common cause of elbow pain, affecting approximately 2% to 3% of the general population and up to 40% of athletes participating in overhead sports, such as tennis.[1,2] A recent large-scale, population-based study estimated that nearly 1 million individuals in the United States develop lateral epicondylitis each year.[3] In 80% to 90% of patients, the condition is self-limiting and resolves within a year. Walker-Bone and colleagues,[4] however, found that 27% of patients with lateral epicondylitis had severe difficulties with activities of daily living, and the current consensus is that a year is too long for the patient to wait for relief from pain, disability, and loss of economic productivity.

PATHOLOGY

Generally, lateral epicondylitis results from microtrauma to the extensor carpi radialis brevis, but may involve other tendons within the forearm extensor muscles, such as the extensor digitorum communis.[5] Nirschl described four stages based on severity of tendon involvement: (1) initial inflammatory reaction, (2) angiofibroblastic degeneration, (3) structural failure or rupture, and (4) structural failure plus fibrosis and calcification.[6,7] Most patients who present with sports-related lateral epicondyitis have stage 2 involvement (angiofibroblastic degeneration).

PATIENT EVALUATION/EXAMINATION

The most common complaint of patients with lateral epicondylitis is pain around the bony prominence of the lateral epicondyle that radiates along the forearm within the area of the common extensor mass. Typically, pain is exacerbated by repetitive activities that involve contraction of the forearm extensors.[8] Nirschl

---

The authors have nothing to disclose.
Department of Orthopaedic Surgery & Biomedical Engineering, University of Tennessee-Campbell Clinic, 1211 Union Avenue, Suite 510, Memphis, TN 38104, USA
* Corresponding author.
E-mail address: murphysteiner@gmail.com

described seven stages based on pain severity (Table 1).[6]

NONOPERATIVE TREATMENT

Traditional nonoperative methods include rest, nonsteroidal anti-inflammatory drugs (NSAIDs), bracing, and physical therapy. Because of reports in the literature that corticosteroid injections, although they provide short-term pain relief, may actually have deleterious effects,[9,10] efforts have increased to evaluate biologics that may enhance healing of the degenerated extensor tendons.

Autologous Blood Injection

Autologous whole blood injections (ABI) have been widely used for treatment of lateral epicondylitis. The rationale is that ABI can initiate an inflammatory reaction around the tendon, which leads to cellular and humoral mediators to induce a healing cascade.[11] Another hypothesis is that ABI allows delivery of growth factors that increase vascularity and new collagen formation.[12] In studies comparing ABI with corticosteroids or platelet-rich plasma (PRP), results have been mixed (Table 2).

Two recent meta-analyses came to contradictory conclusions. Tsikopolous and colleagues[14] determined that ABI provides significant clinical relief at 8 to 24 weeks, whereas Sirico and colleagues[13] concluded that currently available data offer no support for the effect of ABI in medium- or long-term follow-up. Several studies found better pain relief at 4 weeks with corticosteroid injections but better long-term results with ABI,[15,20,21] whereas others found ABI more effective at short-term follow-up[19] and others found no differences at either short-term or long-term follow-up.[22,23] Based on their systematic review and network meta-analysis, Arirachakaran and colleagues[17] concluded that, when comparing ABI, PRP, and corticosteroid injections, PRP was best at reducing pain, whereas ABI was best for functional improvements; however, ABI had the highest risk of adverse effects (injection site pain and skin reaction).

Technique (Calandruccio)

A total of 2 mL of autologous blood are drawn from the ipsilateral upper extremity and mixed with 1 mL of 2% lidocaine HCl or 1 mL of 0.5% bupivacaine HCl. The needle is introduced proximal to the lateral epicondyle along the supracondylar ridge and gently advanced into the undersurface of the extensor carpi radialis brevis while infusing the blood-anesthetic mixture extra-articularly (Fig. 1).

A removable 40-degree orthoplast cock-up splint is applied. NSAIDs are withheld, and patients are restricted from using straps, braces, or physiotherapy. At 3 weeks, an interval wrist motion program consisting of stretching the musculature about the wrist and elbow, especially the forearm extensor compartment, is begun. At 6 weeks, patients are released to activities as tolerated.

Platelet-Rich Plasma

PRP has been used extensively in the treatment of tendon, ligament, muscle, bone, and cartilage pathology. It is attractive because it is can be exogenously applied to various tissues, where it releases high concentrations of platelet-derived growth factors that enhance wound healing, bone healing, and tendon healing,[24] in addition to possessing antimicrobial properties that may help prevent infections.[25,26] The major components of PRP are transforming growth factor-β, platelet-derived insulin-like growth factor, insulin-like growth factor, vascular endothelial growth factor, and fibroblast growth factor-2. Transforming growth factor-β1, insulin-like growth factor-1, and platelet-derived insulin-like growth factor stimulate proliferation of mesenchymal cells; in particular, transforming growth factor-β1 stimulates extracellular matrix production, including collagen.[27]

Studies of the clinical efficacy of PRP report varied outcomes (Table 3). In a systematic review, de Vos and colleagues[44] concluded that there is

Table 1 Seven stages of pain severity described by Nirschl	
Phase 1	Mild pain with exercise, resolves within 24 h
Phase 2	Pain after exercise, exceeds 48 h
Phase 3	Pain with exercise, does not alter activity
Phase 4	Pain with exercise, alters activity
Phase 5	Pain with heavy activities of daily living
Phase 6	Pain with light activities of daily living, intermittent pain at rest
Phase 7	Constant pain at rest, disrupts sleep

Adapted from Nirschl RP. Elbow tendinosis/tennis elbow. Clin Sports Med 1992;11:855.

Table 2
Results from studies comparing ABI with corticosteroids or PRP

Author/Date	Compared with	# Patients	Results
Sirico et al,[13] 2016	CC	Meta-analysis	Currently available data offer no support for the effectiveness of ABI in medium- and long-term follow-up.
Tsikopoulos et al,[14] 2016	CC	Meta-analysis	ABI provided significant clinical relief of epicondylopathy at 8–24 wk.
Qian et al,[15] 2016	CC	Meta-analysis	CSIs were more effective than ABIs for pain relief in the short term; however, in the intermediate term, ABIs exhibited a better therapeutic effect for pain relief. ABIs seemed to be more effective at restoring function in the intermediate term.
Chou et al,[16] 2016	CC, PRP	Meta-analysis	ABI more effective than steroid injection, but not more effective than PRP.
Arirachakaran et al,[17] 2016	CC, PRP	Meta-analysis	Both ABI and PRP can improve pain and function; ABI has higher risk of complications.
Arik et al,[18] 2014	CC	80	ABI was more effective in improving pain, function, and grip strength. It is recommended as a first-line injection treatment because it is simple, cheap, and effective.
Jindal et al,[19] 2013	CC	50	ABI was more effective than steroid injection in the short-term follow-up in tennis elbow.
Dojode,[20] 2012[a]	CC	60	The corticosteroid injection group showed a statistically significant decrease in pain compared with ABI group in visual analogue scale and Nirschl stage at 1 wk and at 4 wk. At the 12-wk and 6-mo follow-up, the ABI group showed statistically significant decrease in pain compared with corticosteroid injection group. At the 6-month final follow-up, a total of 14 patients (47%) in the corticosteroid injection group and 27 patients (90%) in ABI group were completely relieved of pain.
Ozturan et al,[21] 2010	CC ECSWT	60	Corticosteroid injection gave significantly better results for all outcome measures at 4 wk; success rates in the three groups were 90%, 16.6%, and 42.1%, respectively. ABI and ECSWT gave significantly better Thomsen provocative test results and upper extremity functional scores at 52 wk; the success rate of corticosteroid injection was 50%, which was significantly lower than the success rates for ABI (83.3%) and ECSWT (89.9%). Corticosteroid injection provided a high success rate in the short term. However, ABI and ECSWT gave better long-term results, especially considering the high recurrence rate with corticosteroid injection. Authors suggested that the treatment of choice for lateral epicondylitis is ABI.
Wolf et al,[22] 2011	CC, saline	28	No differences in DASH scores at 2- and 6-mo follow-up. All three groups had improved outcomes at 6 mo.
Stenhouse et al,[23] 2013	Dry needling	28	Trend toward greater clinical short-term improvement with ABI, but no significant difference demonstrated at each follow-up interval.

[a] Prospective, randomized trial; CC, corticosteroid; CCI, corticosteoid injection; DASH, Disabilities of the Arm, Shoulder, and Hand; ECSWT, extracorporeal shock wave therapy.

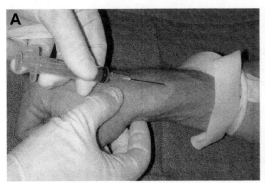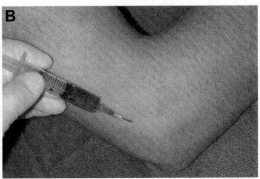

Fig. 1. (*A*) A total of 2 mL of autologous blood drawn from the dorsal vein of the hand. (*B*) Introduction of the needle proximal to the lateral epicondyle along the supracondylar ridge and advanced into the undersurface of the extensor carpi radialis. (*From* Edwards SG, Calandruccio JH. Autologous blood injections for refractory lateral epicondylitis. J Hand Surg 2003;28(2):274; with permission.)

Table 3
Varied outcomes reported from studies of the clinical efficacy of PRP

Author/ Date	Compared with	# Patients	Results
Karaduman et al,[28] 2016	Surgery	110	PRP found to be superior for pain relief and function in short- and mid-term follow-up.
Palacio et al,[29] 2016	CC	60	No evidence that one treatment was more effective than another.
Montalvan et al,[30] 2016	Saline	50	PRP injections were not more efficacious than saline injections.
Khaliq et al,[31] 2015	CC	102	Corticosteroids effective in 53%, PRP effective in 82% at 3-wk follow-up.
Yadav et al,[32] 2015	CC	65	PRP-treated group showed significantly better improvement compared with corticosteroid group at 3-mo follow-up.
Lebiedzinski et al,[33] 2015	CC	99	At 6 wk and 6 mo, mean DASH score was significantly better in steroid group, but better in PRP group at 1 y. Steroids gave more rapid improvement, but therapeutic effect is longer lasting in PRP group.
Ford et al,[34] 2015	Surgery	78	Similar outcomes in pain improvement and return to work.
Behera et al,[35] 2015	Bupivacaine	25	Improvement in scores was greater in PRP group after 3 mo; differences in scores between groups were significant at 6 mo and 1 y: VAS 83% vs 46%, modified Mayo score 47% vs 21%, Nirschl score 77% vs 56%.
Gautam et al,[36] 2015	CC	30	PRP seemed to enable biologic healing of the lesion; steroids seemed to provide short-term, symptomatic relief but resulted in tendon degeneration.
Raeissadat et al,[37] 2014	ABI	76	Both treatments were effective at all time points for 12-mo follow-up.

Author/ Date	Compared with	# Patients	Results
Mishra et al,[38] 2014	Active controls	230	Success rates at 12 wk were 75% for PRP vs 66% for control; at 24 wk, success rates were 84% for PRP vs 68% for active control subjects.
Tonk et al,[39] 2014	Low-level laser	81	Mean Nirschl pain score decreased significantly from baseline with PRP compared with low-level laser therapy.
Krogh et al,[40] 2013	CC, saline	60	Neither injection of PRP nor steroid was superior to saline with regard to pain reduction at 3 mo.
Thanasas et al,[41] 2011	ABI	28	Greater VAS score improvement with PRP at every follow-up interval, but statistically significant only at 6 wk.
Gosens et al,[42] 2011	CC	100	PRP more frequently improved DASH and VAS than did steroid. At 2 y, scores returned to baseline for the steroid group but remained improved for PRP group.
Creaney et al,[12] 2011	ABI	150	66% success in PRP group vs 72% in ABI group; higher rate of conversion to surgery in ABI group (20%) vs PRP group (10%).
Peerbooms et al,[43] 2010	CC	100	Pain reduction and improved function in PRP group exceeded those in CC group.

Abbreviation: VAS, visual analogue scale.

strong evidence that PRP injections are not effective in treating chronic lateral epicondylitis. Several studies have shown that PRP is not more effective than corticosteroid injections or ABI or even saline,[29,30,34,37,40] whereas others have reported better pain relief and function with PRP.[38,41–43]

PRP solutions can vary from patient to patient, with the device used to prepare it, the time and method of storage before use, injection technique, and the addition of other materials or biologics. The concentration of platelets in PRP can vary from 2.5 to 9 times that of normal blood (150,000–450,000 platelets per microliter). The ideal level of platelet concentration for PRP injection has not been determined. One laboratory study suggested that a concentration of 2.5 times that of normal blood was ideal and that higher concentrations might actually limit new cell growth.[45] Current recommendations are that the platelet concentration be raised to four to six times above the baseline concentration.[46] The concentration of white blood cells also is controversial; some experts believe that white blood cells inhibit the healing response,[47] whereas others think they have no negative or beneficial effects.

Cited contraindications to PRP injection include hematologic blood dyscrasias with platelet dysfunction; septicemia or fever; cutaneous infections in the area to be injected; anemia (hemoglobin <10 dL); malignancy, particularly with hematologic or bony involvement; and allergy to bovine products if bovine thrombus is to be used.[46]

Before PRP injections patients are required to refrain from the use of corticosteroids and NSAIDs for 2 to 3 weeks, discontinue anticoagulation use 5 days before the procedure, and increase fluid intake in the 24 hours before the procedure.[46]

Technique (Martinez)

Various centrifuge systems are commercially available. Blood is drawn from a vein (typically 15–50 mL) and processed in the centrifuge machine. Bovine thrombin and/or calcium may be used as an activation agent, depending on the procedure, and bupivacaine and/or epinephrine may be added. Ultrasound is used to guide needle placement. After a local anesthetic is injected, a small amount of PRP (often 3–6 mL) is injected into the joint capsule and a bandage is applied. After the injection, patients are kept supine for 15 minutes to allow binding of the PRP to the tendon. A home-based stretching and strengthening program is begun 48 hours after injection, and full return to activity is allowed as tolerated.

SUMMARY

Most patients are able to avoid surgery for lateral epicondylitis with the use of non-operative management techniques, but the course of recovery can be prolonged and frustrating for some patients. Orthobiologics, such as autologous blood and PRP injections, have the potential to improve pain and function in a shorter time frame. While the results of current literature can be confusing and contradictory, many studies have demonstrated their efficacy. More research is needed to determine how to best use orthobiologics in the treatment of lateral epicondylitis.

REFERENCES

1. Verhaar JA. Tennis elbow. Anatomical, epidemiological and therapeutic aspects. Int Orthop 1994; 18:263–7.
2. Shiri R, Viikari-Juntura E, Varonen H, et al. Prevalence and determinants of lateral and medial epicondylitis: a population study. Am J Epidemiol 2006;164:1065–74.
3. Sanders TL Jr, Maradit Kremers H, Bryan AJ, et al. The epidemiology and health care burden of tennis elbow: a population-based study. Am J Sports Med 2015;43:1066–71.
4. Walker-Bone K, Palmer KT, Reading D, et al. Occupation and epicondylitis: a population-based study. Rheumatology (Oxford) 2012;51(2):305–10.
5. Kraushaar BS, Nirschl RP. Tendinosis of the elbow (tennis elbow). Clinical features and findings of histological, immunohistochemical, and electron microscopy studies. J Bone Joint Surg Am 1999;81:259–78.
6. Nirschl RP. Prevention and treatment of elbow and shoulder injuries in the tennis player. Clin Sports Med 1988;7:289–308.
7. Nirschl RP, Pettrone FA. Tennis elbow. The surgical treatment of lateral epicondylitis. J Bone Joint Surg Am 1979;61:832–9.
8. Calfee RP, Patel A, DaSilva MF, et al. Management of lateral epicondylitis: current concepts. J Am Acad Orthop Surg 2008;16(1):19–29.
9. Bisset L, Smidt N, van der Windt DA, et al. Conservative treatments for tennis elbow—do subgroups of patients respond differently? Rheumatology 2007;46:1602–5.
10. Smidt N, van der Windt DA, Assendelft WJ, et al. Corticosteroid injections, physiotherapy, or a wait-and-see policy for lateral epicondylitis: a randomised controlled trial. Lancet 2002;359:657–62.
11. Edwards SG, Calandruccio JH. Autologous blood injections for refractory lateral epicondylitis. J Hand Surg Am 2003;28:272–8.
12. Creaney L, Wallace A, Curtis M, et al. Growth factor-based therapies provide additional benefit beyond physical therapy in resistant elbow tendinopathy: a prospective, single-blind, randomised trial of autologous blood injections versus platelet-rich plasma injections. Br J Sports Med 2011;45:966–71.
13. Sirico F, Ricca F, Di Meglio F, et al. Local corticosteroid versus autologous blood injections in lateral epicondylitis: meta-analysis of randomized controlled trials. Eur J Phys Rehabil Med 2016. [Epub ahead of print].
14. Tsikopoulos K, Tsikopoulos A, Natsis K. Autologous whole blood or corticosteroid injections for the treatment of epicondylopathy and plantar fasciopathy? A systematic review and meta-analysis of randomized controlled trials. Phys Ther Sport 2016;22:114–22.
15. Qian X, Lin Q, Wei K, et al. Efficacy and safety of autologous blood products compared with corticosteroid injections in the treatment of lateral epicondylitis: a meta-analysis of randomized controlled trials. PM R 2016;8:780–91.
16. Chou LC, Liou TH, Kuan YC, et al. Autologous blood injection for treatment of lateral epicondylosis: a meta-analysis of randomized controlled trials. Phys Ther Sport 2016;18:68–73.
17. Arirachakaran A, Sukthuayat A, Sisayanarane T, et al. Platelet-rich plasma versus autologous blood versus steroid injection in lateral epicondylitis: systematic review and network meta-analysis. J Orthop Traumatol 2016;17(2):101–12.
18. Arik HO, Kose O, Guler F, et al. Injection of autologous blood versus corticosteroid for lateral epicondylitis: a randomised controlled study. J Orthop Surg (Hong Kong) 2014;22:333–7.
19. Jindal N, Gaury Y, Banshiwal RC, et al. Comparison of short term results of single injection of autologous blood and steroid injection in tennis elbow: a prospective study. J Orthop Surg Res 2013;8:10.
20. Dojode CM. A randomised control trial to evaluate the efficacy of autologous blood injection versus local corticosteroid injection for treatment of lateral epicondylitis. Bone Joint Res 2012;1:192–7.
21. Ozturan KE, Yucel I, Cakici H, et al. Autologous blood and corticosteroid injection and extracorporeal shock wave therapy in the treatment of lateral epicondylitis. Orthopedics 2010;33:84–91.
22. Wolf JM, Ozer K, Scott F, et al. Comparison of autologous blood, corticosteroid, and saline injection in the treatment of epicondylitis: a prospective, randomized, controlled multicenter study. J Hand Surg Am 2011;35:1269–72.
23. Stenhouse G, Sookur P, Watson M. Do blood growth factors offer additional benefit in refractory lateral epicondylitis? A prospective, randomized pilot trial of dry needling as a stand-alone procedure versus dry needling and autologous conditioned plasma. Skeletal Radiol 2013;42:1515–20.

24. Sampson S, Gerhardt M, Mandelbaum B. Platelet rich plasma injection grafts for musculoskeletal injuries: a review. Curr Rev Musculoskelet Med 2008;1:165–74.

25. Foster TE, Puskas BL, Mandelbaum BR, et al. Platelet-rich plasma: from basic science to clinical applications. Am J Sports Med 2009;37:2259–72.

26. Moojen DJ, Everts PA, Schure RM, et al. Antimicrobial activity of platelet-leukocyte gel against Staphylococcus aureus. J Orthop Res 2008;26:404–10.

27. Boyan BD, Schwartz Z, Patterson TE, et al. Clinical use of platelet-rich plasma in orthopaedics. AAOS Now, September 2007.

28. Karaduman M, Okkaoglu MC, Sesen H, et al. Platelet-rich plasma versus open surgical release in chronic tennis elbow: a retrospective comparative study. J Orthop 2016;13:10–4.

29. Palacio EP, Schiavetti RR, Kanematsu M, et al. Effects of platelet-rich plasma on lateral epicondylitis of the elbow: prospective randomized controlled trial. Rev Bras Ortop 2016;51:90–5.

30. Montalvan B, Le Goux P, Kouche S, et al. Inefficacy of ultrasound-guided local injections of autologous conditioned plasma for recent epicondylitis: results of a double-blind placebo-controlled randomized clinical trial with one-year follow-up. Rheumatology (Oxford) 2016;55:279–85.

31. Khaliq A, Khan I, Inam M, et al. Effectiveness of platelets rich plasma versus corticosteroids in lateral epicondylitis. J Pak Med Assoc 2015;65(11 Suppl 3):S100–4.

32. Yadav R, Kothari SY, Borah D. Comparison of local injection of platelet rich plasma and corticosteroids in the treatment of lateral epicondylitis of the humerus. J Clin Diagn Res 2015;9:RC05–7.

33. Lebiedzinski R, Synder M, Buchcic P, et al. A randomized study of autologous conditioned plasma and steroid injections in the treatment of lateral epicondylitis. Int Orthop 2015;39:2199–203.

34. Ford RD, Schmitt WP, Lineberry K, et al. A retrospective comparison of the management of recalcitrant lateral elbow tendinosis: platelet-rich plasma injections versus surgery. Hand (N Y) 2015;10:285–91.

35. Behera P, Dhillon M, Aggarwal S, et al. Leukocyte-poor platelet-rich plasma versus bupivacaine for recalcitrant lateral epicondylar tendinopathy. J Orthop Surg (Hong Kong) 2015;23:6–10.

36. Gautam VK, Verma S, Batra S, et al. Platelet-rich plasma versus corticosteroid injection for recalcitrant lateral epicondylitis: clinical and ultrasonographic evaluation. J Orthop Surg (Hong Kong) 2015;23:1–5.

37. Raeissadat SA, Rayegani SM, Hassanabadi H, et al. Is platelet-rich plasma superior to whole blood in the management of chronic tennis elbow: one year randomized clinical trial. BMC Sports Sci Med Rehabil 2014;6:12.

38. Mishra AK, Skrepnik NV, Edwards SG, et al. Efficacy of platelet-rich plasma for chronic tennis elbow: a double-blind, prospective, multicenter, randomized controlled trial of 230 patients. Am J Sports Med 2014;42:463–7.

39. Tonk G, Kumar A, Gupta A. Platelet rich plasma versus laser therapy in lateral epicondylitis of elbow. Indian J Orthop 2014;48:390–3.

40. Krogh TP, Fredberg U, Stengaard-Pedersen K, et al. Treatment of lateral epicondydlitis with platelet-rich plasma, glucocorticoid, or saline: a randomized, double-blind, placebo-controlled trial. Am J Sports Med 2013;41:625–35.

41. Thanasas C, Papadimitriou G, Charalambidis C, et al. Platelet-rich plasma versus autologous whole blood for the treatment of chronic lateral elbow epicondylitis: a randomized controlled clinical trial. Am J Sports Med 2011;39:2130–4.

42. Gosens T, Peerbooms JC, van Laar W, et al. Ongoing positive effect of platelet-rich plasma versus corticosteroid injection in lateral epicondylitis: a double-blind randomized controlled trial with 2-year follow-up. Am J Sports Med 2011;39:1200–8.

43. Peerbooms JC, Sluimer J, Bruijn DJ, et al. Positive effect of an autologous platelet concentrate in lateral epicondylitis in a double-blind randomized controlled trial: platelet-rich plasma versus corticosteroid injection with a 1-year follow-up. Am J Sports Med 2010;38:225–62.

44. de Vos RJ, Windt J, Wier A. Strong evidence against platelet-rich plasma injections for chronic lateral epicondylar tendinopathy: a systematic review. Br J Sports Med 2014;48:953–6.

45. Graziani F, Ivanovski S, Cei S, et al. The in vitro effect of different PRP concentrations on osteoblasts and fibroblasts. Clin Oral Implants Res 2006;17:212–9.

46. Martinez SF. Practical guidelines for using PRP in the orthopaedic office. AAOS Now September 2010.

47. McCarrel TN, Minas T, Fortier LA. Optimization of leukocyte concentration in platelet-rich plasma for the treatment of tendinopathy. J Bone Joint Surg Am 2012;94:e143(1-8).

Foot and Ankle

Osseous Healing in Foot and Ankle Surgery with Autograft, Allograft, and Other Orthobiologics

Jane C. Yeoh, MD, FRCSC, Brandon A. Taylor, MD*

KEYWORDS

- Bone - Autograft - Allograft - Orthobiologic - Nonunion - Foot - Ankle

KEY POINTS

- In the surgical treatment of foot and ankle abnormality, many problems require bone grafting for successful osseous union.
- Nonunion, reconstruction, and arthrodesis procedures pose specific challenges due to bony defects secondary to trauma, malunions, or previous surgery.
- Nonunion in foot and ankle arthrodesis is a significant risk and is well documented in recent literature.
- This article is a review of the recent literature regarding the use of bone graft and orthobiologics in foot and ankle surgery.

Bone grafting is a common component of foot and ankle surgery that requires successful osseous union. Nonunion, reconstruction, and arthrodesis procedures may pose specific challenges, including bony defects secondary to trauma, malunions, or previous surgery. The average nonunion rate is 10% for ankle arthrodesis[1] and 16% for subtalar joint arthrodesis.[2] Nonunion rates in foot and ankle arthrodesis literature range from 0% to 47%[3] in complex and revision procedures.

In primary arthrodesis of the ankle and hindfoot, the following have been found to increase the risk of nonunion and other noninfectious complications:

- Positive smoking history[2,3]
- Previous attempted fusion[2]
- Presence of avascular bone[2]
- Diabetes mellitus[3]
- Previous solid organ transplantation[3]
- Poor preoperative serum glucose control (>200 mg/dL)[3]

In revision arthrodesis, neuropathy and prior revision attempts have been identified as statistically significant risk factors for nonunion.[4]

Autologous bone grafting (ABG) is the gold standard because of its osteoconductive, osteoinductive, and osteogenic properties. The disadvantages of autograft include limitations in quantity, donor site morbidity, and infections and complications from donor site harvest. For example, one study quoted that 8.8% of patients undergoing autograft procedures have more clinically significant donor site pain (≥20 mm on the visual analogue scale [VAS]) 1 year postoperatively.[5] A recent survey of orthopedic surgeons showed when considering graft for foot and ankle arthrodesis procedures, the strongest factors supporting the use of ABG were clinical or radiographic nonunion, avascular necrosis, smoking history, and evidence of potential for incongruous apposition of bone.[6]

In foot and ankle surgery, many of these clinical scenarios are common, and the surgeon must weigh the advantages and disadvantages

This author has no commercial or financial conflicts or disclosures.
Campbell Clinic Foot & Ankle Department, 1400 South Germantown Road, Germantown, TN 38138, USA
* Corresponding author.
E-mail address: btaylor@campbellclinic.com

when choosing autograft, allograft, and/or orthobiologic bone graft substitute. Orthobiologic bone graft substitutes include cellular bone allograft with mesenchymal stem cells (CBA with MSCs), platelet-derived growth factor (PDGF), platelet-rich plasma (PRP), bone morphogenetic proteins (BMPs), and fetal tissues. This article reviews the various bone grafting and bone substitute options and presents available and recent evidence supporting their use in procedures requiring osseous healing in foot and ankle surgery.

AUTOLOGOUS BONE GRAFTING

ABG continues to be the gold standard because of its osteoinductive, osteoconductive, and osteogenic properties. Harvest from the calcaneus or distal tibial metaphysis can provide small amounts of autograft with minimal complexity added to the procedure. Ipsilateral iliac crest bone graft (ICBG), when harvested as a tricortical wedge, has the added benefit of improved osteoconduction or mechanical support, especially in the setting of an opening wedge osteotomy or large bony defects.

A recent logistic regression analysis of 159 foot and ankle studies from 1959 to 2012 concluded that there is a trend toward higher healing rates when using cancellous and structural ABG in foot and ankle surgery compared with allograft, but this was not statistically significant.[7] However, 153 of 159 studies included in this analysis were retrospective case series. Retrospective case series have inherent methodological limitations and have potential for selection bias. In these retrospective case series, surgeons could have elected the use of their preferred graft for procedures they deemed more complex, or those that had an anticipated lower rate of union. By introducing this variable, the results in these studies may not give an accurate picture of treatment efficacy.

Surgeons may choose to use the reamer-irrigator-aspirator (RIA, DePuy Synthes, West Chester, PN, USA) to collect cancellous ABG from the patient's femoral shaft. Although there is strong evidence supporting RIA use in the orthopedic trauma literature, there is a paucity of data supporting its use in foot and ankle surgery. In 2014, a retrospective study was performed comparing clinical and radiographic outcomes in patients undergoing tibiotalar arthrodesis.[8] When compared with ICBG, use of the RIA showed significantly lower nonunion rates. Furthermore, no patient undergoing RIA had chronic pain at the harvest site compared with 2 in the ICBG

group. Length of stay and radiographic fusion were similar in both groups. The RIA may be a viable alternative to ICBG, especially in terms of reducing nonunion rates and donor site morbidity.

ALLOGRAFT

Allogenic bone grafts (allografts) are harvested from cadavers, avoiding the complications associated with ABG donor site harvest. Although allograft can have osteoconductive properties as does ABG, processing cadaver allograft tissue takes its toll. Although gamma-irradiation and heat sterilization processing are necessary to allow successful transfer of tissue from donor to host, these processes kill live bone cells and cause allograft to lose a significant amount of its osteogenic properties.[9] Processing the graft limits cell viability, which increases osteoblast apoptosis. Graft Processing also destroys other cells that produce cytokines, bone morphogenic proteins, which decreases the osteogenic and osteoinductive properties of the graft. Demineralized bone matrix (DBM) is a form of allograft prepared by acid extraction so it retains BMPs and bone collagens. Therefore, DBM has improved osteoinductive capacity compared with traditional allograft, because it retains more bone morphogenic proteins and bone collagens.[10]

CELLULAR BONE ALLOGRAFT CONTAINING MESENCHYMAL STEM CELLS

CBA containing MSCs is a biologic allograft alternative to traditional ABG and other bone graft substitutes. Like ABG, cadaveric CBA with MSCs have osteoconduction, osteoinduction, and osteogenesis properties. Human undifferentiated MSCs and MSCs differentiated into bone, cartilage, and adipose escape a host's immune system because they express HLA class I, and not HLA class II.[11] Therefore, MSCs from an allogenic or cadaveric source avoids the host's cell-mediated immune response by avoiding the T cells and lymphocyte cell response.[11] Allograft tissue is harvested to preserve living MSCs or osteoprogenitor cells. Processing and specifications of different CBA with MSCs products vary by company and product.

Jones and colleagues[12] conducted a prospective, multicenter trial of cryopreserved CBA with MSCs (Trinity Evolution; Orthofix, Inc, Lewisville, TX, USA) in patients undergoing ankle and/or hindfoot arthrodesis. Trinity Evolution describes a screening process whereby only 3% of cadaveric donors are used and cryopreserves tissue at −185°C. Orthofix assures a minimum of 250,000 living cells per cubic centimeter, 50,000 of which are MSCs or osteoprogenitor cells.[12] In Trinity Evolution, demineralized cortical bone from the same donor is added to the cancellous bone with cellular component.[12] Jones and colleagues[12] enrolled 103 patients with 171 joint arthrodeses; 76 patients with 129 arthrodeses completed the 1-year follow-up. At their primary endpoint 6 months postoperatively, 63 of 92 (69%) patients and 124 of 153 (81%) joints achieved fusion, assessed by plain radiographs and computed tomographic (CT) scan. At 1 year postoperatively, 54 of 76 (71%) patients and 112 of 129 joints (87%) achieved fusion.[12] Patients experienced a statistically significant improvement in clinical outcomes, demonstrated by improved American Orthopaedic Foot and Ankle Society ankle-hindfoot scores, short form-36 physical component score, and VAS compared with baseline.[12]

Anderson and associates[13] performed a retrospective cohort study on 109 consecutive ankle fusions with adjunctive CBA with MSCs compared with proximal tibia ABG. After exclusions, 85 patients remained; 44 patients received CBA with MSCs and 41 patients received proximal tibia bone ABG.[13] The investigators reported that the choice of CBA with MSCs or proximal tibia bone ABG used was determined by patient preference, amount of graft required, and availability of CBA with MSCs.[13] This study did not comment on the specific personal or technical reasons CBA with MSCs or proximal tibia bone ABG was chosen, therefore possibly allowing for selection bias. In addition, the same product of CBA with MSCs was not always used.[13] Anderson and associates[13] published 84% union rate with CBA with MSCs and 95% union rate with ABG, but the difference was not statistically significant (P = .158). However, the group treated with CBA with MSCs had an average time to fusion of 13.0 ± 2.1 weeks compared with 11.0 ± 2.8 weeks in the ABG group (P≤.001). There were no statistically significant differences in complications or patient satisfaction, and no complications occurred related to the proximal tibia ABG donor site.[13]

Protzman and colleagues,[14] Hollawel,[15] Scott and Hyer,[16] and Rush and colleagues[17] each published smaller studies of 25 patients or less examining MSC bone allograft in foot and ankle fusion. These level IV studies demonstrated good and equivocal outcomes. The investigators also published that the CBA with MSCs product was safe and efficacious in foot and ankle arthrodesis.[14,15]

BONE MARROW ASPIRATE

Bone marrow aspirate (BMA) or its concentrate, bone marrow concentrate (BMC), has been used to promote bone repair by delivering pluripotent MSCs to the surgical site while limiting the donor site morbidity associated with ABG. BMA harvest is less invasive than ICBG harvest, and it can be collected under local anesthetic. BMA can enhance bone healing by transplanting stem cells that differentiate into osteoblasts, chondrocytes, and other connective tissue cells.

BMA is often obtained from the ipsilateral iliac crest, long bone metaphyses, or calcaneus. BMA is concentrated to BMC via centrifugation. However, quantitative analysis performed on BMA reveals that some harvest locations have higher concentrations than others. Aspirate obtained from the anterior iliac crest had much higher concentrations of osteoblastic progenitor cells when compared with the aspirate collected from the tibia or calcaneus.[18] Another study comparing the effect of different concentrations of BMC with distal tibia atrophic nonunions found BMC with higher concentrations of progenitor cells were associated with higher rates of bone healing.[19]

Braly and colleagues[20] presented case series evidence showing that BMA is an inexpensive and less invasive therapy for patients with distal tibial metaphyseal nonunions in the setting of stable retained hardware. The patients in this study displayed significant clinical and radiographic improvement from their preintervention state, and 9 of 11 patients attained bony union within 6 months of BMA intervention.

In a case series of zone II and III fifth metatarsal fractures in competitive athletes, Murawski and Kennedy[21] showed that percutaneous screw fixation along with BMC yielded more predictable results in terms of fracture healing. Their mean time to radiographic fracture healing in the BMC treatment group was 5 weeks, and only 2 patients of 26 did not return to their previous level of sporting activity.

BMA has also been useful in the care of diabetic Charcot arthropathy. In 2009, Pinzur[22] presented a case series of 44 patients. Surgical treatment of 46 feet was performed with the use of BMA mixed with PRP. Most of these patients had open wounds with chronic draining osteomyelitis.[22] Forty-two of 46 feet had radiographic evidence of bony fusion at 16 weeks postoperative. These 42 feet also had no drainage or evidence of infection at an average of 26 months after surgery.[22] It is thought that BMA provides the pluripotent cells, and PRP adds cytokines that stimulate healing. PRP will be discussed in further detail later.

PLATELET-DERIVED GROWTH FACTOR

PDGF is a polypeptide growth factor that plays a role in embryogenesis,[23] angiogenesis,[24] and osteogenesis.[25] PDGFs are a family of growth factors, classified in groups A, B, C, and D, that forms heterodimers and homodimers.[24] PDGF is released by platelets and macrophages at the sites of injury, and sites of blood clot and early bone healing.[24] These PDGFs and cytokines have chemoattractant and mitogenic effects, thereby increasing the concentration of additional neutrophil and macrophages to sites of healing.[24] As a result, PDGFs help advance the healing cascade in endochondral ossification.[24]

The homodimeric form of PDGF subunit B is PDGF-BB. PDGF-BB's role in formation, repair, and regeneration of bone has been postulated in the mesengenic process, involving MSCs.[25] PDGF-BB is involved in osteoblastic processes by several mechanisms, including the following:

1. Stimulation of vascular endothelial growth factors (VEGF) by pericytes,
2. Liberating and activating pericytes to functional MSCs,
3. Mitogenic effects for pericytes and MSCs,
4. Affecting other factors involved in osteogenesis, including BMPs,
5. Additional complex communication and coordination functions with PDGF-receptors, MSCs, pericytes, endothelial cells and other signaling pathways.[25]

Another mechanism PDGF-BB indirectly affects osteogenesis is through its role in angiogenesis. PDGF-BB, with the synergistic effect of fibroblastic growth factor-2 (FGF-2), is potently angiogenic and has vascular stabilization effects; this has been demonstrated in the cornea and in hindfoot ischemia of rodents.[26]

Preclinical studies have demonstrated therapeutic value of recombinant human PDGF-BB (rhPDGF-BB) in animals before human use. Initially, rhPDGF-BB benefits were demonstrated in periodontal defects in dogs. Subsequently, rhPDGF-BB studies were performed in osteoporotic fracture models in geriatric rats, fracture healing models in diabetic rats, and distraction osteogenesis models in the femur of rats.[27]

RhPDGF-BB has been studied in several areas of orthopedic surgery, including foot and ankle surgery.[28] RhPDGF-BB is US Food and Drug Administration (FDA) approved for foot and ankle uses and is sold as Regranex (Smith & Nephew, Memphis, TN, USA), which is approved for wound healing in ulcers, Augment Bone Graft (BioMimetic Therapeutics, Franklin, TN, USA), which is approved for foot and ankle arthrodesis, and Augment Injectable Bone Graft (BioMimetic Therapeutics), which is approved for foot and ankle.[28] Augment Injectable Bone Graft is approved for foot and ankle arthrodesis in Canada and is under investigation for this use in the United States.[28]

RhPDGF-BB has been used in combination with β-tricalcium phosphate (β-TCP) carrier. β-TCP is a ceramic bone graft substitute with osteoconductive properties that has been used in orthopedic surgeries before the advent of PDGF.[29] RhPDGF-BB with β-TCP (rhPDGH/β-TCP) is approved for foot and ankle arthrodesis in the United States, Canada, Australia, and New Zealand (Augment Bone Graft; BioMimetic Therapeutics).[28] Before approval of rhPDGF-BB/β-TCP in foot and ankle surgery, rhPDGF-BB/β-TCP was demonstrated in a randomized controlled multicenter trial to be beneficial in periodontal defect surgery.[30] RhPDGF-BB/β-TCP has been compared with ABG in several studies described in later discussion.[5,31–33]

Daniels and colleagues[31] performed a prospective, open-label, Canadian multicenter trial using rhPDGF-BB/β-TCP (Augment Bone Graft; BioMimetic Therapeutics) in 60 patients undergoing midfoot, hindfoot, or ankle arthrodesis. This pilot trial followed 60 patients, 59 of which completed the study to 36 weeks (9 months) with clinical and radiographic assessments. Fifty-two of 59 (88%) patients achieved radiographic union during the study.[31] Overall, 54 of 60 (90%) patients and 124 of 130 (95.4%) joints treated with rhPDGF-BB/β-TCP had clinical success within 12 months.[31] Five of 6 of these patients that did not unite had midfoot nonunions, and the remaining 1 of 6 of the patients with nonunion belonged to the ankle/hindfoot group.[31] Daniels and colleagues[31] were able to demonstrate adequate safety, efficacy, and noninferiority of rhPDGF-BB/β-TCP in ankle, hindfoot, and midfoot fusion and set the stage for following randomized controlled trials.

In 2011, DiGiovanni and colleagues[32] performed a prospective randomized controlled multicenter trial to assess the feasibility of rhPDGF-BB/β-TCP with ABG. This feasibility study enrolled 20 adult patients undergoing ankle or hindfoot fusion at a 2:1 ratio of rhPDGF-BB/β-TCP to ABG. Fourteen patients received rhPDGF-BB/β-TCP (Augment Bone Graft; BioMimetic Therapeutics) with rigid internal fixation compared with 6 patients who received ABG with rigid fixation of their ankle or hindfoot arthrodesis.[32] Nineteen of 20 patients completed the 36-week study.[32] At 36 weeks, 10 of 13 (77%) patients treated with rhPDGF-BB/β-TCP had achieved osseous union, determined by greater than 50% osseous bridging on CT scan.[32] In contrast, 3 of 6 (50%) patients receiving ABG achieved osseous union.[32] Two patients from the rhPDGF-BB/β-TCP group had a nonunion requiring revision.[32] In addition, DiGiovanni and colleagues[32] documented an increase in operative time by 26 minutes in the ABG group.

Following the feasibility trial, DiGiovanni and associates[5] performed a prospective randomized controlled multicenter trial comparing rhPDGF-BB/β-TCP (Augment Bone Graft; BioMimetic Therapeutics) to ABG in patients receiving hindfoot or ankle arthrodesis. This study enrolled 434 patients in 37 centers in the United States and Canada, and 397 patients remained after disqualifying criteria (exclusions, medical issues). Again, the group used the 2:1 ratio, enrolling 260 patients (394 joints) into the rhPDGF-BB/β-TCP group and 137 patients (203 joints) in the ABG group.[5] Following the groups for 52 weeks, DiGiovanni and associates[5] demonstrated comparable fusion rates clinically and radiographically for the most part. Some differences were found in the all-joints analysis (n = 597); the CT-determined fusion rate at 24 week was 66.5% in the rhPDGF-BB/β-TCP group and 62.6% in the ABG group (P<.001).[5] As well, 3-aspect radiographic union at 52 weeks also demonstrated a difference of 48.5% union in the rhPDGF-BB/β-TCP group and 44.3% in the ABG group (P<.001).[5] Clinical healing and pain at the arthrodesis sites were comparable in both groups.[5] ABG patients had more clinically significant donor site pain (≥20 mm on the VAS) at 24 and 52 weeks, respectively.[5] In addition, 1 patient was hospitalized for donor site infection, and 1 patient had donor site cellulitis.[5]

Notably, the investigators reported decreased radiographic union rates in patients receiving greater volumes of rhPDGF-BB/β-TCP graft.[5] When separated into volumes of rhPDGF-BB/β-TCP used (1–3 cc, 4–6 cc, or 7–9 cc), patients receiving 7 to 9 cc had decreased radiographic healing rates, which were comparable to union rates when ABG was used.[5] In a subsequent analysis, DiGiovanni and colleagues[34] determined that adequate graft fill determined by thin-cut CT scans at 9 weeks is an important factor in successful union of ankle and hindfoot fusions.

In 2015, Daniels and associates[33] performed a prospective randomized controlled multicenter study on rhPDGF-BB/β-TCP with type 1 bovine collagen matrix (rhPDGF-BB/β-TCP-collagen) (Augment Injectable Bone Graft; BioMimetic Therapeutics, Inc, now Wright Medical Technologies, Franklin, TN, USA). The injectable rhPDGF-BB in β-TCP-collagen carrier with cannula allows an option for easier handling. This study of 75 patients requiring ankle or hindfoot fusion enrolled 63 patients into the rhPDGF-BB/β-TCP-collagen group and 12 patients into the ABG control group.[33] Daniels and associates[33] used 142 historical control patients from another study by DiGiovanni and colleagues. The investigators documented a clinically significant improved CT-determined fusion rate in the rhPDGF-BB/β-TCP-collagen group of 84.1% compared with 67.0% in the ABG group at 24 weeks (P<.001). Radiographic results generally either favored fusion rates in the rhPDGF-BB/β-TCP-collagen group compared with ABG or trended toward favoring the rhPDGF-BB/β-TCP-collagen group but did not reach statistical significance. In addition, Daniels and associates[33] established that rhPDGF-BB/β-TCP-collagen patients achieved union more quickly, at 14.3 ± 8.9 weeks compared with 19.7 ± 11.5 weeks when ABG was used (P<.001). Both groups had equivocal clinical union rates of 87.3% and 88.3% at 52 weeks with rhPDGF-BB/TCP-collagen and ABG, respectively. There was no statistically significant difference in therapeutic failures (nonunions, delayed union, further surgery).[33] The rhPDGF-BB/transforming growth factor-β (TGF-β)-collagen group experienced improved clinical success rate (weight-bearing VAS and no secondary procedures), and no donor site pain and comorbidities.[33]

PLATELET-RICH PLASMA

PRP is a concentrate obtained by centrifuging a patient's autologous blood.[35] PRP preparations differ by platelet concentration, leukocyte concentration, activation method, centrifugation method, and delivery method.[28] The PRP concentrate, which is a volume of plasma with platelets and growth factors approximately 5 times that of physiologic normal, is then delivered to soft tissues or bony areas to incite healing.[35]

Platelets function to secrete vesicles, or release granules, important to osseous healing.[35] Alpha-granules are particularly important in this process.[35] Once platelets have degranulated, granules release PDGF, TGF-β, epidermal growth factor, insulin-like growth factor, VEGF, serotonin, thrombospondin-1, and basic FGF-2, which have numerous mitogenic, chemotactic, angiogenic, and differentiation functions.[35] MSCs are then stimulated to differentiate into osteoblasts.[35]

The basic science processes of PRP have been demonstrated in vitro. Slater and associates[36] demonstrated dose-dependent increased osteoblast proliferation in vitro in platelet-treated medium compared with serum-free medium or serum supplemented with 10% fetal calf serum. The investigators also demonstrated increased differentiated properties, including matrix formation and mineral deposition, when platelet-treated medium was used.[36] When the platelet-rich medium was added to fetal calf serum, the effect was even greater.[36]

PRP was originally reported in oral and maxillofacial surgery and used in mandibular defects.[37] In a total of 88 patients with mandibular defects >5 cm, the oral surgeons reported grafts with PRP demonstrated radiographic healing and maturation 1.6 to 2.1 times faster than grafts without PRP.[37]

In orthopedics, PRP has been used in soft tissues (tendon, ligaments, and muscles), osseous healing, and osteochondral lesions.[28] More specifically, PRP is used and reported in lateral epicondylitis, patellar tendinopathy, knee osteoarthritis, acute ligamentous injuries, acute muscle injuries, anterior cruciate ligament reconstruction, rotator cuff repair, articular cartilage repair, and to decrease blood loss in total knee arthroplasty in the areas of sports medicine and general orthopedics.[38] In the foot and ankle, PRP has been published in the soft tissue areas of Achilles tendinopathy,[28] plantar fasciitis,[28] and acute Achilles tendon repair.[38] PRP with respect to osseous healing and fusion in foot and ankle surgery is addressed in later discussion.

Bibbo and colleagues[39] prospectively enrolled 62 high-risk patients undergoing 123 ankle, hindfoot, midfoot, or forefoot arthrodesis procedures using PRP combined with ABG or allograft in a single-surgeon study. All patients in this study received PRP concentrate prepared with Symphony I & II Platelet Concentrating System (Depuy Acromed, Raynham, MA, USA). If the patient required bone graft, they received either ABG or allograft if they refused ABG.[39] There was no comparison group that did not receive PRP. Average time to union of all patients was 41 days, and there was a 94% union rate in terms of both fusion sites (116 of 123) and patients (58 of 62).[39] There were 4 of 62 (6.5%) patient or 7 of 123 (6%) fusion site nonunions.[39] Four of 62 (6.5%) patients developed

deep infection.[39] Investigators noted no complications related to collection of autologous blood for PRP.[39] In addition, Bibbo and colleagues[39] conducted a 30-minute dry-run training for teaching the PRP process to operating staff and how to use equipment.

Wei and associates[40] enrolled 254 patients with 276 Sanders type III calcaneus fractures treated with open reduction and internal fixation with a lateral locking plate and either ABG alone, allograft with PRP, or allograft alone. In this study, PRP was prepared with Landesberg protocol and 2 centrifugation cycles using a Centrifuge 9800 (Kubota, Osaka, Japan). The investigators followed patients' clinical outcomes and radiographic outcomes for 72 months.[40] Wei and associates[40] found statistically significant differences in radiographic outcomes between ABG alone and allograft with PRP compared with allograft alone at 24 and 72 months. The investigators reported no statistically significant difference in these results when comparing ABG alone to allograft with PRP. The group did not find any statistically significant difference in residual pain, walking activities, subtalar range of motion, or ankle-hindfoot alignment between any of the 3 groups.[40] The investigators concluded that allograft with PRP is equivalent to ABG and does not involve any issues with donor site morbidity.[40]

Coetzee and colleagues[41] assessed the use of PRP (Symphony PCS; Depuy, Warsaw, IN, USA) in syndesmotic fusion with the Agility (DePuy, Warsaw, IN, USA) total ankle arthroplasty (TAA). The Agility TAA implant has a specific design that incorporates the distal tibiofibular syndesmosis in the tibial component, and the technique necessitates syndesmosis fusion. Coetzee and colleagues[41] compared 2 prospectively collected groups of patients receiving Agility TAA, one group with routine lateral approach syndesmotic preparation and fixation (114 patients) and the second group with the same syndesmotic preparation with added PRP (66 patients). The investigators noted statistically significant lower rates of syndesmotic delayed union or nonunion rates (6% with PRP compared with 26% without PRP) in the group treated with PRP. In addition, there were statistically significant greater union rates at all time frames measured (8 weeks, 12 weeks, and 6 months).[41]

BONE MORPHOGENETIC PROTEINS

BMPs belong to a TGF-β superfamily.[42] BMPs bind to distinct BMP type I and type II receptors and activate an intracellular signal cascade.[42] Activated intracellular transcription dimerizes and translocates to the nucleus, regulating gene transcription in osteoblasts and chondrocytes.[42] Urist[43(p3070)] first described a "morphogenetic matrix or inductive substratum" when the investigator demonstrated de novo bone cell differentiation in tissue culture medium.[43] Urist demonstrated that morphogenetic matrix (decalcified rodent bone matrix) differentiated into new bone when he added minced muscle or plasma to the culture media.

Currently there are more than 20 BMPs known,[42,44,45] with roles in the bone, brain, heart, kidney, skin, and intestines.[42] Seven BMPs play a role in bone formation and bone turnover.[45] rhBMP-2 and rhBMP-7 are FDA approved for orthopedic surgery in spinal fusion, open tibial fractures, and long bone nonunions.[28] rhBMP-2 and rhBMP-7 are currently used off-label in foot and ankle arthrodesis, high-risk fractures, and nonunion procedures.[28]

rhBMP-2 is produced as Infuse (Medtronic, Minneapolis, MN, USA), and rhBMP-7 is also known as Osteogenic Protein-1 (OP-1; Olympus-Biotech; Stryker, Kalamazoo, MI, USA).[28] rhBMP-2 and rhBMP-7 have been studied in foot and ankle fusion and nonunion healing.

Bibbo and colleagues[45] reported 69 high-risk patients (one or more risk factors for nonunion) with 112 fusion sites who received rhBMP-2 on a collagen sponge (Infuse, Medtronic, Memphis, TN, USA) during ankle and hindfoot arthrodesis surgery. These patients were retrospectively reviewed examining fusion rates, clinical outcomes, and complications. One hundred eight of 112 (96%) of patients achieved union.[45] The investigators reported 5 of 112 (4%) joint nonunions or 3 of 69 (4%) patient nonunions.[45] Two of 41 (5%) subtalar joints, 1 of 19 (5%) talonavicular joints, and 1 of 20 (5%) calcaneocuboid joint arthrodesis procedures resulted in nonunion. Six of 69 (8.7%) patients had complications (nonunion or infection).[45] In this study, their nonunion rate was lower than historical comparison.[1,2]

DeVries and associates[46] retrospectively reviewed revision tibiotalocalcaneal (TTC) arthrodesis cases by retrograde intramedullary nail, comparing TTC nails with rhBMP-2 (7 patients) to TTC nails without the use of rhBMP-2 (16 patients). The group treated using TTC nail without BMP also may have received other bone grafting, including BMA, PRP, or other orthobiologic agent.[46] Investigators described the union rates, time to weight-bearing, radiographic outcomes, and complications. The results did not reach statistical significance.[46]

Fourman and associates[47] performed a retrospective cohort review on 96 patients undergoing complex ankle fusion with circular external fixator (Ilizarov or Taylor Spatial Frame, Smith & Nephew, Memphis, TN, USA) with and without rhBMP-2 (Infuse, Medtronic). Patients were considered complex if they had systemic issues (comorbidities) or local issues associated with poor surgical healing. After exclusions, 82 patients remained; the first 40 patients had a complex ankle fusion with external fixation without rhBMP-2 and the latter 42 patients with rhBMP-2.[47] Patients treated with rhBMP-2 (39 of 42, 92%) had statistically significantly higher CT-determined union rates compared with patients treated without rhBMP-2 (21 of 40, 53%) when assessed within 3 months of surgery (P<.001).[47] When final union was assessed in the cohort treated with rhBMP-2 (40 of 42, 92%) compared with or without rhBMP-2 (33 of 40, 82%) at the time of frame removal (regardless of further intervention), the difference between union rates did not reach statistical significance (P = .08).[47] There was no difference in complication rates.[47]

Rearick and associates[48] published a retrospective case series of 48 patients with 51 cases treated with rhBMP-2 (Infuse, Medtronic) in addition to foot and ankle arthrodesis or revision treatment of fracture nonunion. Using plain radiographs, CT if necessary, and clinical assessment, they demonstrated a 92% (47 of 51) case union rate and a 95% (78 of 82) anatomic site union rate. The average time to union was 111 days (95% confidence interval [CI] 101–121).[48] Fourteen of 83 (17%) sites used ABG in addition to rhBMP-2, and 9 of 83 (11%) sites used allograft in addition to rhBMP-2. Rearick and associates[48] discussed that their union rate was similar to that of Bibbo and colleagues,[45] and lower than historical studies.

In 2009, Schuberth and associates[49] retrospectively reported on 35 high-risk patients with 38 cases requiring ankle fusion, TTC fusion, distal tibial osteotomy, or forefoot procedure who received rhBMP-7 (OP-1; Stryker Biotech, Hopkinton, MA, USA) as a part of their procedure. Once broken down into respective groups, the numbers became too small to interpret.[49] The investigators reported 32 of 38 (84%) of procedures had successful union at an average of 14 weeks.[49]

Ristiniemi and colleagues[50] retrospectively reviewed 20 patients with distal tibia fractures (that were deemed too distal for intramedullary nailing) treated with external fixation with rhBMP-7 with bovine carrier (Osigraft; Stryker Biotech, Limerick, Ireland) compared with control. The control group was 20 matched patients who were treated with external fixation without rhBMP-7.[50] They matched the groups by age (within 15 years), gender, fracture type, fracture shape, tibial defect, and diaphyseal extension.[50] Although the investigators demonstrated all fractures in both groups united, there were improved early outcomes in the rhBMP-7 group.[50] More fractures treated with rhBMP-7 achieved union at 16 weeks postoperatively (14 of 20 [70%] patients treated with rhBMP-7 compared with 6 of 20 [30%] control, P = .039).[50] Increased union with rhBMP-7 was also apparent at 20 weeks (16 of 20 [80%] patients treated with rhBMP-7 compared with 8 of 20 [40%] in the control group, P = .022).[50] Use of rH-BMP-7 translated into statistically significant decreased time to union in patients treated with rhBMP-7 (15.7 weeks in patients treated with rhBMP-7 compared with 23.5 weeks in the control group, P = .002), decreased duration in external fixation (15 weeks in patients treated with rhBMP-7 compared with 21.4 weeks in the control group, P = .037), and decreased duration off work (6.3 months in patients treated with rhBMP-7 compared with 9.0 months in the control group, P = .018).[50]

rhBMP-2 has been studied more extensively in orthopedic spine literature than foot and ankle surgery, and the reported complications rhBMP-2 in spine fusion surgery differ from foot and ankle surgery. In spine fusion studies, rhBMP-2 has been shown to be associated with heterotopic ossification, retrograde ejaculation, and an increased risk for cancer.[51] Fu and associates[51] performed a systematic review and meta-analysis of 13 RCTs (n = 1981) and found a total of 17 cases of cancer. The increased risk for cancer when using rhBMP-2 compared with controls showed a relative risk of 3.45 (CI 1.98–6.00) at 24 months, but no increased risk was observed at 48 months.[51] The investigators noted that cancer risk increased at 2 to 4 years, and the cancers reported were heterogeneous.[51] Fu and associates[51] could not conclude if the cancer risk was dose-related. In addition, the investigators discussed that the cases of cancer were likely underreported and the results should be interpreted with care.

FETAL TISSUES

Fetal tissues, or placental membranes, are layered membranes harvested from donor mothers after healthy cesarean sections.[52] The specific structure and biologic composition of fetal tissues permit unique antiscarring, anti-inflammatory, regeneration, and immune-privilege properties.[52] Fetal tissues were used initially in ophthalmology and have been applied in other medical and surgical fields,

including vascular surgery, general surgery, plastic surgery, urologic surgery, obstetrics and gynecology, wound healing, and orthopedic surgery.[52]

Fetal tissues are composed of an inner amniotic membrane (toward fetal tissues) and an outer chorionic membrane (toward maternal tissues).[52] The inner amniotic membrane, which is further divided into an epithelial layer, basement membrane, and stromal layer, is distinct for its healing potential.[52] The outer chorionic membrane, which is further divided into a reticular layer and trophoblastic layer, has villi that function as a barrier between maternal and fetal blood vessels.[52]

Multiple cytokines, growth factors, and matrix proteins contribute to unique properties of fetal tissues. Specifically, interleukin (IL)-10, IL-1 receptor antagonist, tissue inhibitor of metalloproteinase-1, -2, -3, -4, hyaluronic acid (HA), and the stromal layer of the amniotic membrane have antiscarring properties.[52] IL-10 and the suppression of TGF-β signaling are responsible for the anti-inflammatory properties of fetal tissues.[52] Type III and IV collagen, high-molecular-weight HA, and multiple growth factors[52,53] are credited for the unique matrix and regenerative properties of fetal tissues. Low quantities of HLAs allow fetal tissues to be immune privileged during pregnancy and when used as allograft.[52]

Fetal tissues were initially used as fresh grafts.[52] Advancement in preparation, sterilization, and storage allows more widespread use in medicine.[52] Fetal tissue products differ in their processing, and these processes may entail cryopreservation, dehydration, glycerol preservation, lipophilization, gamma irradiation, ethanol sterilization, and silver impregnation.[52]

The use of fetal tissues in foot and ankle abnormalities has been published in human studies and animal models. Foot and ankle abnormalities that have been published include chronic wounds and diabetic foot ulcers, plantar fasciitis, tendon repair, peripheral nerve repair, cartilage healing, and bone healing.[52] To the authors' knowledge, no studies specifically provide evidence supporting the use of fetal tissue in osseous union in human foot and ankle surgery.

Kerimoglu and colleagues[53] compared human amniotic fluid (HAF) at 18 weeks gestation, HAF at the end of gestation, and control (no HAF) in 36 rat tibia and fibula fractures. Using radiologic, scintigraphic, and histologic examination 3 weeks and 5 weeks after fracture, the investigators determined that fracture healing scores were highest in rats treated with HAF collected at 18 weeks' gestation, followed by HAF at the end of gestation, and the controls had the lowest fracture healing scores. The difference scores between all 3 groups were statistically significant.[53]

Karaçal and associates[54] used a rabbit cranial defect model to examine bony healing of defects treated with HAF compared with normal saline control. The HAF was donated at 16 to 20 weeks' gestation. Ten rabbits were each administered HAF at the cranium defect on one side and normal saline at the cranial defect on the contralateral side.[54] The defects were then examined radiographically using CT scan 3, 4, 5, and 6 weeks postoperatively, and histologically 6 weeks postoperatively.[54] Defects that were treated with HAF had more ossification both radiographically and histologically compared with control.[54]

SUMMARY

Although the literature presented may suggest that achieving osseous union in foot and ankle surgeries is more reliable through the addition of bone grafting procedures and orthobiologic products, the investigators believe higher level evidence is still required to better support their use. There is limited evidence for the use of orthobiologics in osseous union in foot and ankle surgery. It is imperative to continue producing evidence to demonstrate that these interventions will provide better outcomes, fewer complications, and fewer subsequent procedures for surgical patients. Furthermore, with rising costs of health care and emphasis on quality-based reimbursement for physicians, surgeons must be able to justify using extra procedures and adjuvant products. Researchers and health care providers should aspire to provide high-quality evidence, ideally prospective randomized controlled trials, to enhance the knowledge in bone grafting and orthobiologics in foot and ankle surgery as well as in orthopedics in general.

REFERENCES

1. Haddad SL, Coetzee JC, Estok R, et al. Intermediate and long-term outcomes of total ankle arthroplasty and ankle arthrodesis, a systematic review of the literature. J Bone Joint Surg Am 2007;89-A(9):1899–905.
2. Easley ME, Trnka H, Schon LC, et al. Isolated subtalar arthrodesis. J Bone Joint Surg Am 2000;82-A(5):613–24.
3. Myers TG, Lowery NJ, Frykberg RG, et al. Ankle and hindfoot fusions: comparison of outcomes in patients with and without diabetes. Foot Ankle Int 2012;33(1):20–8.
4. O'Connor KM, Johnson JE, McCormick JJ, et al. Clinical and operative factors related to successful revision arthrodesis in the foot and ankle. Foot Ankle Int 2016;37(8):809–15.
5. DiGiovanni CW, Lin SS, Baumhauer JF, et al. Recombinant human platelet-derived growth factor-BB and beta-tricalcium phosphate (rhPDGF-BB/b-TCP): an alternative to autogenous bone graft. J Bone Joint Surg Am 2013;95-A(13):1184–92.
6. Baumhauer JF, Pinzur MS, Daniels TR, et al. Survey on the need for bone graft in foot and ankle fusion surgery. Foot Ankle Int 2013;12:1629–33.
7. Lareau CR, Deren ME, DiGiovanni CW, et al. Does autogenous bone graft work? A logistic regression analysis of data from 159 papers in the foot and ankle literature. Foot Ankle Surg 2015;3:150–9.
8. Nodzo SR, Kaplan NB, Hohman DW, et al. A radiographic and clinical comparison of reamer-irrigator-aspirator versus iliac crest bone graft in ankle arthrodesis. Int Orthop 2014;6:1199–203.
9. Nguyen H, Morgan DA, Forwoo MR. Sterilization of allograft bone: effects of gamma irradiation on allograft biology and biomechanics. Cell Tissue Bank 2007;8(2):93–105.
10. Flynn JM. Orthopaedic knowledge update 10. In: Lu C, Meinberg E, Marcucio R, et al, editors. Fracture repair and bone grafting. 10th edition. Rosemont (IL): AAOS; 2011. p. 11–21.
11. Le Blanc K, Tammik C, Rosendahl K, et al. HLA expression and immunologic properties of differentiated and undifferentiated mesenchymal stem cells. Exp Hematol 2003;31(10):890–6.
12. Jones CP, Loveland J, Atkinson BL, et al. Prospective, multicenter evaluation of allogeneic bone matrix containing viable osteogenic cells in foot and/or ankle arthrodesis. Foot Ankle Int 2015;36(10):1129–37.
13. Anderson JJ, Boone JJ, Hansen M, et al. Ankle arthrodesis fusion rates for mesenchymal stem cell bone allograft versus proximal tibia autograft. J Foot Ankle Surg 2014;53(6):683–6.
14. Protzman NM, Galli MM, Bleazey ST, et al. Biologic augmentation of foot and ankle arthrodeses with an allogeneic cancellous sponge. Orthopedics 2014;37(3):e230–6.
15. Hollawel SM. Allograft cellular bone matrix as an alternative to autograft in hindfoot and ankle fusion procedures. J Foot Ankle Surg 2012;51(2):222–5.
16. Scott RT, Hyer CF. Role of cellular allograft containing mesenchymal stem cells in high-risk foot and ankle reconstructions. J Foot Ankle Surg 2013;52(1):32–5.
17. Rush SM, Hamilton GA, Ackerson LM. Mesenchymal stem cell allograft in revision foot and ankle surgery: a clinical and radiographic analysis. J Foot Ankle Surg 2009;48(2):163–9.

18. Hyer CF, Berlet GC, Bussewitz BW, et al. Quantitative assessment of the yield of osteoblastic connective tissue progenitors in bone marrow aspirate from the iliac crest, tibia, and calcaneus. J Bone Joint Am Surg 2013;95:1312–6.

19. Hernigou P, Poignard A, Beaujean F, et al. Percutaneous autologous bone-marrow grafting for nonunion. Influence of the number and concentration of progenitor cells. J Bone Joint Am Surg 2005; 87:1430–7.

20. Braly HL, O'Connor DP, Brinker MR. Percutaneous autologous bone marrow injection in the treatment of distal meta-diaphyseal tibial nonunions and delayed unions. J Orthop Trauma 2013;9:527–33.

21. Murawski CD, Kennedy JG. Percutaneous internal fixation of proximal fifth metatarsal Jones fractures (zones II and III) with Charlotte Carolina screw and bone marrow aspirate concentrate: an outcome study in athletes. Am J Sports Med 2011;6:1295–301.

22. Pinzur MS. Use of platelet-rich concentrate and bone marrow aspirate in high-risk patients with Charcot arthropathy of the foot. Foot Ankle Int 2009;30:124–7.

23. Alvarez RH, Kantarjian HM, Cortes JE. Biology of platelet-derived growth factor and its involvement in disease. Mayo Clin Proc 2006;81(9):1241–57.

24. Hollinger JO, Hart CE, Hirsch SN, et al. Recombinant human platelet-derived growth factor: biology and clinical applications. J Bone Joint Surg Am 2008;90(Suppl 1):48–54.

25. Caplan AI, Correa D. PDGF in bone formation and regeneration: new insights into a novel mechanism involving MSCs. J Orthop Res 2011;29:1795–803.

26. Cao R, Bråkenhielm E, Rawliuk R, et al. Angiogenic synergism, vascular stability and improvement of hind-limb ischemia by a combination of PDGF-BB and FGF-2. Nat Med 2003;9(5):604–13.

27. DiGiovanni CW, Lin S, Pinzur M. Recombinant human PDGF-BB in foot and ankle fusion. Expert Rev Med Devices 2012;9(2):111–22.

28. Lin SS, Montemurro NJ, Krell ES. Orthobiologics in foot and ankle surgery. J Am Acad Orthop Surg 2016;24(2):113–22.

29. Liu B, Lun D. Current application of β-tricalcium phosphate composites in orthopaedics. Orthop Surg 2012;4(3):139–44.

30. Nevins M, Giannobile WV, McGuire MK, et al. Platelet-derived growth factor stimulates bone fill and rate of attachment level gain: results of a large multicenter randomized controlled trial. J Periodontol 2005; 76(12):2205–15.

31. Daniels T, DiGiovanni C, Lau JT, et al. Prospective clinical pilot trial in a single cohort group of rhPDGF in foot arthrodeses. Foot Ankle Int 2010; 31(6):473–9.

32. DiGiovanni CW, Baumhauer J, Lin SS, et al. Prospective, randomized, multi-center feasibility trial of rhPDGF-BB versus autologous bone graft in a foot and ankle fusion model. Foot Ankle Int 2011; 32(4):344–54.

33. Daniels TR, Younger AS, Penner MJ, et al. Prospective randomized controlled trial of hindfoot and ankle fusions treated with rhPDGF-BB in combination with a β-TCP-collagen matrix. Foot Ankle Int 2015;36(7):739–48.

34. DiGiovanni CW, Lin SS, Daniels TR. The importance of sufficient graft material in achieving foot and ankle fusion. J Bone Joint Surg Am 2016;98-A(15): 1260–7.

35. Bibbo C, Hatfield S. Platelet-rich plasma concentrate to augment bone fusion. Foot Ankle Clin N Am 2010;15:641–9.

36. Slater M, Patava J, Kingham K, et al. Involvement of platelets in stimulating osteogenic activity. J Orthop Res 1995;13(5):655–63.

37. Marx RE, Carlson ER, Eichstaedt RM, et al. Platelet-rich plasma, growth factor enhancement for bone grafts. Oral Surg Oral Med Oral Pathol Oral Radiol Endod 1998;85(6):638–46.

38. Foster TE, Puskas BL, Mandelbaum MB, et al. Platelet-rich plasma: from basic science to clinical applications. Am J Sports Med 2009;37(11): 2259–72.

39. Bibbo C, Bono CM, Lin SS. Union rates using autologous platelet concentrate alone and with bone graft in high-risk foot and ankle surgery patients. J Surg Orthop Adv 2005;14(1):17–22.

40. Wei LC, Lei GH, Sheng PY, et al. Efficacy of platelet-rich plasma combined with allograft bone in the management of displaced intra-articular calcaneal fractures: a prospective cohort study. J Orthop Res 2012;30(10):1570–6.

41. Coetzee JC, Pomeroy GC, Watts JD, et al. The use of autologous concentrated growth factors to promote syndesmosis fusion in the agility total ankle replacement. A preliminary study. Foot Ankle Int 2005;26(10):840–6.

42. Abe E. Function of BMPs and BMP antagonists in adult bone. Ann N Y Acad Sci 2006;1068:41–53.

43. Urist M. The classic, a morphogenetic matrix for differentiation of bone tissue. Clin Orthop Relat Res 2009;467(12):3068–70. Reprint from: Urist M. A morphogenetic matrix for differentiation of bone tissue. Calcif Tissue Res 1970;Suppl:98–101.

44. El-Amin SF, Hogan MV, Allen AA, et al. The indications and use of bone morphogenetic proteins in foot, ankle, and tibia surgery. Foot Ankle Clin N Am 2010;15:543–51.

45. Bibbo C, Patel DV, Haskell MD. Recombinant bone morphogenetic protein-2 (rhBMP-2) in high-risk ankle and hindfoot fusions. Foot Ankle Int 2009; 30(7):597–603.

46. DeVries JG, Nguyen M, Berlet GC, et al. The effect of recombinant bone morphogenetic protein-2 in

revision tibiotalocalcaneal arthrodesis: utilization of the retrograde arthrodesis intramedullary nail database. J Foot Ankle Surg 2012;51(4):426–32.

47. Fourman MS, Borst EW, Bogner E, et al. Recombinant human BMP-2 increases the incidence and rate of healing in complex ankle arthrodesis. Clin Orthop Relat Res 2014;472(2):732–9.

48. Rearick T, Charlton TP, Thordarson D. Effectiveness and complications associated with recombinant human bone morphogenetic protein-2 augmentation of foot and ankle fusions and fracture nonunions. Foot Ankle Int 2014;35(8):783–8.

49. Schuberth JM, DiDomenico LA, Mendicino RW. The utility and effectiveness of bone morphogenetic protein in foot and ankle surgery. J Foot Ankle Surg 2009;48(3):309–14.

50. Ristiniemi J, Flinkkilä T, Hyvönen P, et al. RhBMP-7 accelerates the healing in distal tibial fractures treated by external fixation. J Bone Joint Surg Br 2007;89(2):265–72.

51. Fu R, Selph S, McDonagh M, et al. Effectiveness and harms of recombinant human bone morphogenetic protein-2 in spine fusion, a systematic review and meta-analysis. Ann Intern Med 2013;158(12):890–902.

52. Hanselman AE, Lalli TA, Santrock RD. Use of fetal tissue in foot and ankle surgery. Foot Ankle Spec 2015;8(4):297–304.

53. Kerimoglu S, Livaoglu M, Sönmex B, et al. Effects of human amniotic fluid on fracture healing in rat tibia. J Surg Res 2009;152(2):281–7.

54. Karaçal N, Kosocu P, Çobanglu Ü, et al. Effect of human amniotic fluid on bone healing. J Surg Res 2005;129(2):283–7.

Restorative Tissue Transplantation Options for Osteochondral Lesions of the Talus: A Review

John Chao, MD[a],*, Andrew Pao, MD[b]

KEYWORDS

- Osteochondral lesion of talus • Osteochondral allograft • Osteochondral autologous transplant
- DeNovo • PRP

KEY POINTS

- Larger osteochondral lesions of the talus greater than 1.5 cm^2 have increased risk for healing complications.
- Osteochondral autograft transfer improves functional outcomes and pain scores in medium to short-term periods.
- Most of the success rate of osteochondral allografts is based on retrospective case series with limited outcome data.
- Autologous chondrocyte implantation has been shown to improve American Orthopedic Foot and Ankle Society scores but most studies do not correlate results with specific characteristics of the lesion.
- There are limited clinical data to support the use of platelet rich plasma, hyaluronic acid, bone marrow aspirate concentrate, or juvenile cartilage for osteochondral lesions of the talus.

INTRODUCTION

Osteochondral lesions of the talus (OLTs) are more common than previously thought. They are associated with trauma and are frequently involved in patients presenting with ankle sprains or fractures. The range of OLTs occurring after ankle trauma has been reported to be between 10% and 75%.[1–4]

Diagnosis can be difficult because plain radiographs may miss more than half of osteochondral lesions.[5] On clinical examination, there is not a specific test that is diagnostic for osteochondral lesion of the talus. Patients may present with diffuse nonspecific tenderness, or the pain may be more specific over the medial or lateral talus. Computed tomography (CT) and MRI are frequently used for the evaluation of suspected OLT. MRI is typically preferred for assessing the integrity of the overlying cartilage in nondisplaced lesions. CT scans are better at showing cystic lesions that may be overestimated with the edema seen on MRI. In addition, CT scans have been reported to be more accurate at determining lesion size.[6]

Various classification schemes have been devised, with some based on radiographic findings and some based on intraoperative arthroscopic findings regarding the condition of the osteochondral fragment. The Berndt and Harty classification is based on plain radiography (Box 1), the Hepple classification is based on MRI, and the Ferkel and Sgaglione classification is based on CT scan.[7,8]

The authors have nothing to disclose.
[a] Peachtree Orthopaedic Clinic, 5505 Peachtree Dunwoody Road, Suite 600, Atlanta, GA 30342, USA; [b] Atlanta Medical Center, 303 Parkway Drive, Northeast, Atlanta, GA 30312-1212, USA
* Corresponding author.
E-mail address: jchao@pocatlanta.com

Arthroscopic treatment of osteochondral lesions has been associated with worse outcomes for large cystic lesions. Shoulder lesions of the talus are also challenging because the curved geometry is hard to reproduce. Uncontained osteochondritis dissecans (OCD) of the talar shoulder have more complicated clinical outcomes than those with a contained nonshoulder lesion.[12] In these cases, restorative tissue transplantation options include use of autograft, allograft, autologous chondrocyte implantation (ACI), and juvenile cartilage allograft transplantation. This article focuses on these transplantation options and seeks to provide an up-to-date evidence-based summary of the literature.

After diagnosis of a symptomatic OLT, initial treatment is nonoperative. This may include anti-inflammatories, immobilization, and protected weightbearing. The main contraindication to nonoperative treatment is an acute injury with displacement. In these cases, prompt operative management is indicated to either resect or perform reduction and internal fixation of the fragment.[9]

Surgical intervention is indicated for the remainder of osteochondral lesions that have failed conservative management. Bony or ligament reconstruction may also be necessary at time of surgery. Ankle arthroscopy is the most common treatment modality for OLT. Often, the osteochondral lesion is treated with debridement or marrow stimulation. Penetration of the subchondral plate leads to release of mesenchymal stem cells and growth factors that forms a clot that develops into fibrocartilage. This type-I collagen has different biomechanical properties than native articular hyaline cartilage, which is composed primarily of type-II collagen. Debridement and marrow stimulation have been well reported in the literature and shown to be effective for lesions less than 1.5 cm^2.[10] This cutoff of 1.5 cm^2 is based on several prior studies, and lesion size has been accepted widely as the most commonly used predictor of clinical outcomes after bone marrow stimulation for OLT. However, recent literature has failed to detect a significant correlation between lesion size and clinical outcomes after bone marrow stimulation.[11] In fact, a recent systematic review found that lesion sizes greater than 107.4 mm^2 and 10.2 mm in diameter are significantly correlated with poorer clinical outcomes.[11] The investigators reported that the variability in calculating lesion size area makes the current cutoff of 1.5 cm^2 inaccurate.

OSTEOCHONDRAL AUTOGRAFT TRANSPLANTATION SYSTEM

Osteochondral autograft transplantation system (OATS) involves harvesting cylindrical blocks of cartilage and bone from a donor site such as

- Trochlea and sulcus terminalis of the ipsilateral knee
- Superolateral aspect of the lateral femoral condyle (**Fig. 1**)
- Ipsilateral distal tibia
- Ipsilateral talus.

Although osteochondral autologous transplantation has traditionally been used as salvage for failed primary treatment, its use as the primary procedure has been supported by several studies. Benefits of OATS allows for bony healing with hyaline cartilage and no concern for an immune response destroying the graft. Disadvantages include donor site morbidity and

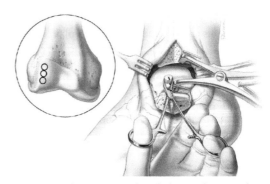

Fig. 1. Autologous osteochondral transplantation harvested from the knee. One or more cylindrical grafts are transplanted into the talar lesion, taking care to keep the articular surface congruent. (*From* Murawski CD, Kennedy JG. Operative treatment of osteochondral lesions of the talus. J Bone Joint Surg Am 2013;95(11):1049; with permission.)

the possible need for an osteotomy to expose the lesion. Nonunion and delayed union of the osteotomy is reported to occur at a rate between 0% and 2%.[13] Because OATS is more common in the knee, it is not uncommon to request the help of a knee surgeon who can help with harvest of the graft.

Gobbi and colleagues[14] performed a randomized controlled trial comparing outcomes of chondroplasty versus microfracture versus osteochondral autologous transplantation in subjects with symptomatic OLTs. Mean time to follow-up was 53 months. Mean lesion size ranged from 3.7 cm² to 4.5 cm². OATS was shown to have similar outcome scores when compared with chondroplasty and microfracture at 2-year follow-up. American Orthopedic Foot and Ankle Society (AOFAS) scores were 85 in 12 subjects with grade 3 or 4 lesions treated with autograft taken from the ipsilateral knee. However, the OATS group had significantly higher numeric pain intensity scores postoperatively when compared with the other 2 modalities. The investigators recommended chondroplasty or microfracture as first-line surgical treatment of patients with OLT.

Multiple studies have investigated the use of OATS for OLT. Most demonstrate improvement in AOFAS score and low incidence of complication (Table 1).

Multiple studies have evaluated donor-site knee pain after osteochondral graft harvest. Although there are some data on poorer results in patients with increased body mass index, most data reports a relatively low incidence of morbidity with good clinical scores.[28,29]

The ability of patients to return to sporting activities has also been studied. Paul and colleagues[30] studied 131 subjects who were followed retrospectively for a mean of 60 months postoperatively after autologous osteochondral transplantation. Although subjects were able to return to sporting activities, there was a reduction of participation in high-impact and contact sports. The investigators also noted that both the surgical site and donor site morbidity could contribute to reduction in sporting activities due to concern about an excessive load or the risk of trauma to the ankle or the morbidity of the graft harvest at the knee.

OATS may also be done for revision OCD surgery. One study showed that primary OATS show better functional outcomes versus secondary OATS after failed microfracture. Their cohort consisted of 22 subjects with primary and 54 subjects with secondary OATS. The postoperative Foot and Ankle Outcome Score (FAOS) was 10 points higher in the primary group.[31]

OSTEOCHONDRAL ALLOGRAFT TRANSPLANTATION

Osteochondral allograft transplantation is more frequently used when the OLT is too large to fill with autograft. It is a single-stage procedure in which a cadaver graft of viable articular cartilage and underlying subchondral bone are matched to the osteochondral defect. Fresh allografts are typically preferred due to decreased chondrocyte viability in the donor tissue having been reported in both fresh-frozen and cryopreserved allografts.[32,33] Due to allografts being hypothermically stored for a minimum of 14 days as a result of safety concerns over infection and viability of chondrocytes having been shown to decrease after 28 days postmortem, it is recommended that the fresh osteochondral allografts be used between 15 and 28 days postmortem, ideally at day 15 to 16 to maximize chondrocyte viability.[34] Fig. 2 shows allograft harvest and fixation to talus.

The biggest advantage is that it easier to match the unique shape of the talus with the allograft. Disadvantages include

- Limited availability of graft because the patient and surgeon must wait for a size-matched talus
- Time-sensitive nature of surgery because the fresh allograft should be implanted 14 to 21 days after harvest
- Concerns of disease transmission or immunologic factors.

Donors are screened for diseases such as human immunodeficiency virus, hepatitis, prion disease, and syphilis. Regarding immunologic factors, Pomajzl and colleagues[35] reported on 8 failed allografts and thought that biologic causes were likely responsible for failure. They suspected possible CD4+ and CD8+ lymphocyte-mediated failure.

Fresh allografts are the most commonly used in practice and the literature on osteochondral allografts mostly comprises retrospective studies. When interpreting the data, one must remember than allograft is typically used on larger lesions with more cystic characteristics. Table 2 shows studies looking at allograft transplant of talar OCD.

Ahmad and Jones[44] looked at 40 subjects using either autograft from the ipsilateral distal femoral condyle or allograft for recurrent or large OLTs. Mean size of the autograft and allograft group was 1.6 cm² and 1.8 cm², respectively. Autograft had a decrease of visual analog scale (VAS) from 7.9 to 2.2, whereas the

Table 1
Studies investigating the use of osteochondral autograft transplantation system for osteochondral lesions of the talus

Study	Number of Subjects	Follow-up	Donor Site	Outcome	Results
Sammarco & Makwana,[15] 2002	12	25 mo	Talus	AOFAS improved from 64 to 90	AOFAS scores higher in subjects <40 y All subjects very satisfied No donor site complications
Emre et al,[16] 2012	32	24 mo	Knee	AOFAS improved from 59 to 88	Open mosaicplasty is reliable for OCD with subchondral cysts >1.5 cm diameter
Imhoff et al,[17] 2011	26	84 mo	Knee	AOFAS improved from 50 to 78 VAS decreased from 7.8 to 1.5	Normal integration of transplant on MRI did better OATS as a 2nd procedure had worse clinical AOFAS and higher VAS
Hu et al,[18] 2013	16	32.6 mo	Iliac crest	VAS decreased from 5.5 to 1 AOFAS improved from 75 to 90	7 subjects resumed sporting activities 7 excellent, 8 good, and 1 fair results
Kim et al,[19] 2012	52	13.1 mo	Knee	AOFAS improved from 67 to 83 VAS improved from 6.9 to 3.3	1 required scope 13 mo later with soft tissue impingement
Hintermann et al,[20] 2015	14	4.1 y	Knee	AOFAS increased from 65 to 81 VAS decreased from 5.8 to 1.8	Vascularized bone graft from femur can restore contour of talus
Chen et al,[21] 2015	15	24 mo	Talus	AOFAS increased from 49 to 89 VAS decreased from 5 to 1 MOCART was 64	Autograft from medial tibia can treat large cystic OCD lesions
de l'Escalopier et al,[22] 2015	37	76 mo	Knee	AOFAS postoperatively was 83 Work-related accident related with poorer result	Mosaicplasty gives good midterm outcomes in 78%
Scranton & McDermott,[23] 2001	50	36 mo	Knee	90% with good to excellent score 1 subject with impingement that improved after release	Cystic stage V lesion can be treated with OATS

Study	Number of Subjects	Follow-up	Donor Site	Outcome	Results
Kreuz et al,[24] 2006	35	49 mo	Talus	AOFAS improved by 39 points without osteotomy and 30 points with osteotomy. No nonunions of osteotomy	Tibial wedge osteotomy is good alternative for malleolar osteotomy
Lee et al,[25] 2003	17	36 mo	Knee	89% excellent and 11% good results. Second-look arthroscopy in 16 ankles revealed congruity in 88%	OATS can treat advanced-stage OCD of talus
Al-Shaikh et al,[26] 2002	19	16 mo	Knee	AOFAS postoperatively score was 88. Lysholm knee score was 97. 2 with mild knee pain	OATS effective for salvage surgery
Flynn et al,[27] 2016	85	47 mo clinical 25 mo MRI	Knee	FAOS improved from 50 to 81	OATS effective for large OCLs of the talus and MOCART scoring indicated good structural integrity of the graft

Abbreviations: FAOS, Foot and Ankle Outcome Score; MOCART, magnetic resonance observation of cartilage repair tissue; VAS, visual analog scale.

allograft group had a decrease of VAS from 7.8 to 2.7. However, 3 subjects had symptomatic nonunion and 2 were converted to OATS from the ipsilateral distal femoral condyle. The investigators concluded that, although results for allograft were comparable to autograft, fresh talar allograft may have lower healing rates than autograft.

COMBINED ALLOGRAFT-AUTOGRAFT

Zhu and Xu[45] reported on osteochondral autograft transfer combined with cancellous allograft as a treatment of large cystic talar osteochondral lesions. Twelve subjects, all with defects larger than 15 mm in diameter, were available for follow-up at a mean of 25.4 months. The cyst was filled with cancellous allograft and the autograft plug was placed on top of it. AOFAS scores improved from 64 to 88 and VAS decreased from 6 to 1. Seven subjects rated their result as excellent and 5 as good. At the follow-up of 18 months postoperatively, no subjects had knee complaints. Two subjects had mild stiffness of the ankle but all subjects had returned to work at the latest 6 months after surgery.

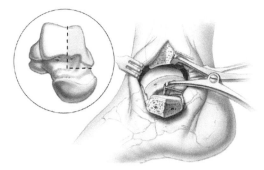

Fig. 2. Osteochondral allograft harvested from size-matched talus is transplanted into the prepared talus and secured using internal fixation. (*From* Murawski CD, Kennedy JG. Operative treatment of osteochondral lesions of the talus. J Bone Joint Surg Am 2013;95(11):1050; with permission.)

Table 2
Studies investigating allograft transplant of talar osteochondritis dissecans

Study	Number of Subjects	Follow-up	Outcome	Conclusion
Gross et al,[36] 2001	9	12 y	3 required fusion due to resorption and fragmentation of graft Average survival of 9 grafts was 9 y	Results are promising
Raikin,[37] 2009	15	54 mo	AOFAS improved from 38 to 83 VAS improved from 8.5 to 3.3 5 rated result as excellent, 6 as good, 2 as fair, and 2 as poor 2 ankles converted to fusion at 32 and 76 mo postoperatively	Bulk fresh osteochondral allograft is viable option
Görtz et al,[38] 2010	12	38 mo	Mean Olerud-Molander Ankle Score improved from 28 to 71 Overall graft survival rate 10/12 Of surviving grafts, 3/10 rated excellent, 2/10 good, 3/10 fair, 2/10 poor 9/10 satisfied	Significant improvement in function and pain with good subject satisfaction
Hahn et al,[39] 2010	13	48 mo	AOFAS score improved from 45 to 81 Foot Function Index improved from 5.56 to 2.01 All subjects reported ability to return to daily activities within a year of surgery	Reasonable procedure for younger subjects with focal osteochondral talar defects
El-Rashidy et al,[40] 2011	38	38 mo	AOFAS improved from 52 to 79 VAS decreased from 8.2 to 3.3 15 postoperative MRIs showed minimal graft subsidence and articular congruence Graft failure in 4 subjects	Fresh osteochondral allograft is effective
Adams et al,[41] 2011	8	48 mo	VAS decreased from 6 to 1 Postoperative AOFAS score was 84 Mean Lower Extremity Functional Scale improved from 37 to 65	Midterm results in fresh allograft transplant can be successful in large OCD of talar shoulder
Haene et al,[42] 2012	17	4.1 y	AOFAS hindfoot scores were collected only postoperatively (average 79) Osteolysis (n = 5), subchondral cysts (n = 8), and degenerative changes (n = 7)	High reoperation rate 2 grafts did not incorporate 5 ankles considered failures
Orr et al,[43] 2016	8	28.5 mo	AOFAS score improved from 49.6 to 73 Mean pain VAS improved from 6.9 to 4.5	Modest improvement in short-term functional outcome scores

AUTOLOGOUS CHONDROCYTE IMPLANTATION

ACI is a 2-stage procedure in which chondrocytes are harvested from the patient and grown in culture. The first-generation of this procedure involved using an autologous periosteal flap to seal the implanted cell bed. However, due to concerns with periosteal patch hypertrophy causing increased reoperation rates, most ACI procedures are now performed using a hyaluronan, porcine collagen, and bovine collagen scaffold.[46] **Fig. 3** shows the 2 stages of ACI.

A newer variation of this technique, matrix ACI (MACI) is based on the same principle but the chondrocytes are implanted on a collagen matrix. To the authors' knowledge, ACI for the talus is considered investigational because only ACI for the knee has been approved by the US Food and Drug Administration (FDA). MACI for the knee has just been approved to be done in the United States in December 2016 by the FDA.

There is a lack of controlled studies comparing ACI with other methods of cartilage repair. There are several retrospective studies that have reported improvements with ACI or MACI (**Table 3**).

AUTOLOGOUS MATRIX-INDUCED CHONDROGENESIS

Autologous matrix-induced chondrogenesis is a single-step procedure that involves debridement of the cartilage lesion, microfracture, and placement of an acellular collagen matrix sealed with fibrin glue. Because OLTs are typically associated with large cystic osseous lesions, some investigators have modified the existing technique by adding autologous iliac crest cancellous bone to reconstruct the bony defect underneath the cartilage.[56]

Valderrabano and colleagues[56] showed that use of autologous matrix-induced chondrogenesis

was a viable option. Iliac crest was grafted into talar defect and an acellular collagen matrix was placed on top and sealed with fibrin glue. Subjects had increased AOFAS scores from 60 to 89 postoperatively with decrease in VAS from 5 to 1.6. Magnetic resonance observation of cartilage repair tissue (MOCART) score for cartilage repair on postoperatively MRI averaged 62. The investigators had complete filling in 35% but with hypertrophic cartilage in 50%. The number of subjects that participated in sports increased from 12% to 62%.

Wiewiorski and colleagues[57] reported on autologous matrix-induced chondrogenesis also. They reported on 60 subjects at a mean of 47 months follow-up. VAS improved from 6.9 to 2.3. Their cohort participated at a similar low postoperative sports and recreational activity level compared with preoperative levels.

JUVENILE CARTILAGE ALLOGRAFT TRANSPLANTATION

The use of particulated juvenile allograft cartilage (PJAC) is a newer technique for osteochondral lesion of the talus. Because it is a preparation of immature articular cartilage, PJAC contains a much higher cellular density when compared with mature articular cartilage.[58] The juvenile cartilage is inserted into the defect and sealed with fibrin glue (**Fig. 4**).

Advantages of this technique include being a single-stage procedure with no donor site morbidity. Juvenile chondrocytes have shown superior capability to provide the cushioning properties for cartilage.[58] Examples of PJAC that have been developed include BioCartilage (Arthrex, Cartilage Extracellular Matrix) and DeNovo NT (Zimmer, particulated juvenile cartilage).

BioCartilage contains desiccated, particulated allograft cartilage that is hydrated with platelet-rich plasma and placed into cartilage defects in which microfracture has been

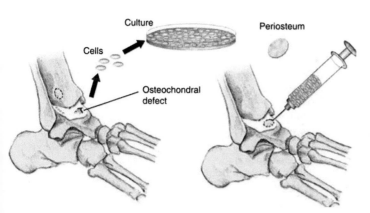

Fig. 3. The first procedure of ACI is harvest of cartilage cells from the talus. These cells are grown in culture. These cultured cells are transplanted into the OCD underneath a periosteal patch removed from tibia. (*From* Mitchell ME, Giza E, Sullivan MR. Cartilage transplantation techniques for talar cartilage lesions. J Am Acad Orthop Surg 2009;17(7):411; with permission.)

Table 3
Retrospective studies reporting improvements with autologous chondrocyte implantation or matrix autologous chondrocyte implantation

Study	Number of Subjects	Follow-up	Outcome	Conclusion
Giannini et al,[47] 2009	10	10 y	AOFAS improved from 38 to 92 MRI showed well-modeled articular surface Regenerated cartilage showed no significant difference compared with healthy hyaline cartilage	ACI in ankle comparable with the knee
Giannini et al,[48] 2008	46	12 and 36 mo	AOFAS score improved from 57 to 86.8 (12 mo) and 89.5 (36 mo) Histologic examination showed hyaline cartilage regeneration	Excellent clinical and histologic results of ACI
Giannini et al,[49] 2014	46	87 mo	AOFAS score improved from 57 to 92 3 failures	Arthroscopic ACI to repair osteochondral lesions of talus can have good outcomes
Lee et al,[50] 2011	21	1 y	Follow-up MRI and second-look arthroscopy performed 1-y postoperatively	Second-look arthroscopy not necessary after ACI as MRI is good for evaluating postoperatively
Nam et al,[51] 2009	11	38 mo	AOFAS score improved from 47 to 84 10 underwent second-look arthroscopy with complete coverage of defect seen in all subjects	ACI yields significant functional improvement for talar OCD
Kwak et al,[52] 2014	29	70 mo	No correlation found between lesion size and follow-up AOFAS score 24 underwent postoperative MRI 22 demonstrated 75% repair tissue fill 2 demonstrated 50%–75% repair tissue fill	Improvement in all parameters tested with enduring long-term results in subjects
Baums et al,[53] 2007	12	63 mo	AOFAS score improved from 44 to 88 MRI showed nearly congruent joint surface in 7 subjects, discrete irregularities in 4, and incongruent surface in 1	Promising clinical results of ACI
Schneider & Karaikudi,[54] 2009	20	21 mo	AOFAS score improved from 60 to 87 Significant overall improvement in pain scores	MACI is reliable treatment of talar osteochondral defects (mean size 233 mm^2)
Giza et al,[55] 2010	10	1 and 2 y	AOFAS scores improved from 61 to 74 (1 y) and 73 (2 y) SF-36 demonstrated improvement at both 1 and 2 y	MACI may be effective way to treat full-thickness lesions of talus

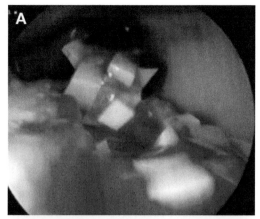

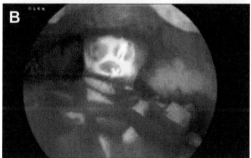

Fig. 4. (A) The particulated juvenile cartilage is placed into a large medial osteochondral lesion of the talus. (B) Graft is sealed with fibrin glue. (*From* Wodicka R, Ferkel E, Ferkel R. Osteochondral lesions of the ankle. Foot Ankle Int 2016;37(9):1031; with permission.)

performed. There are scant papers on its use in equine knees and tibial plafond.[59,60] Currently, to the knowledge of the authors, there are no clinical papers that report on the use of Bio-Cartilage (Arthrex) allograft for talar OCD lesions.

DeNovo is a cartilaginous tissue graft, obtained from juvenile allograft donors up to 13 years old but typically younger than 2 years old. It is provided as particulated tissue pieces each having a volume of approximately 1 mm^3.[58]

There is variability in the treatment of the cystic component of an OCD when using DeNovo because some surgeons have used it in conjunction with either marrow abrasion or bone grafting. A case using DeNovo in which the subject was pain-free at 2 year follow-up has been reported.[61]

In a larger study, Coetzee and colleagues[62] treated 24 ankles in 23 subjects with arthroscopy and DeNovo NT. Fourteen of the ankles had failed after at least 1 prior bone marrow stimulation procedure. Eighteen ankles had at least 1 concomitant procedure performed. Subjects had an average OCD lesion size of 125 plus or

minus 75 mm^2 with average depth of 7 plus or minus 5 mm. All lesions had 1 dimension greater than or equal to 10 mm. Only 6 lesions were fully contained. Follow-up was 16 months, and no postoperative scores were reported because some data was collected retrospectively. AOFAS scores at final follow-up were 85 but were seen to have better results in smaller lesions. There was 92% good or excellent result in lesions between 10 to 15 mm and 56% good or excellent results with lesions greater than 15 mm. The 12-item Short-Form Health Survey (SF-12) physical scores were 46 and mental health was 55. One subject had graft delamination and at revision allograft 25% of grafts had failed to attach to the bone.

Lanham and colleagues[63] evaluated the outcomes of iliac crest bone marrow aspirate (ICBMA) concentrate or collagen scaffold and particulated juvenile articular cartilage for larger articular cartilage lesions of the talus in 12 subjects. Mean lesion size was 1.9 to 2.0 cm^2. AOFAS, Foot and Ankle Ability Measure (FAAM), and SF-12 outcome scores were collected for each subject, with a mean follow-up of 5 months. The investigators concluded that PJAC yielded better clinical outcomes at 2 years when compared with ICBMA.

BIOLOGIC ADJUNCTS

Multiple biologic adjuncts have been used in addition to marrow stimulation. Some of these options include ultrasound stimulation, hyaluronic acid treatment, platelet-rich plasma (PRP), and bone marrow aspirate concentrate (BMAC). The literature is extremely sparse for data supporting the clinical efficacy of these treatments.

PRP has been used both operatively and nonoperatively to treat OCD lesions of the talus. Mei-Dan and colleagues[64] looked the response of talar OCD lesions to a series of 3 injections of hyaluronic acid (weekly) or PRP (biweekly), and concluded that the subjects with PRP did significantly better. Lesion size for the hyaluronate and PRP groups was 1.26 cm^2 and 1.41 cm^2, respectively. The investigators advocated for PRP as first-line nonoperative treatment of these lesions, unless there are definite indications for surgery.

Gormeli and colleagues[65] did a similar study but supplemented microfracture with an intra-articular injection of either hyaluronic acid or PRP. Thirteen subjects received PRP and 14 received hyaluronic acid. Although both groups improved, subjects who received PRP had statistically significant increases in AOFAS scores and decreases in VAS scores compared with hyaluronic acid.

Guney and colleagues[66] reported on 16-month follow-up for marrow stimulation versus stimulation plus PRP and noted the addition of PRP lead to better outcomes in AOFAS and VAS scores. Guney and colleagues[67] reported 42-month follow-up on marrow stimulation versus stimulation plus PRP versus OATS. They concluded that all groups had significant improvements in AOFAS and VAS pain scores, and OATS had significantly better VAS scores versus marrow abrasion.

BMAC has not been used as a stand-alone treatment of OLT. However, it has been used to augment other procedures and has shown promising results. Gianni and colleagues[68] treated OCD lesions greater than 1.5 cm^2 with less than 5 mm depth with debridement and filled the lesion with a mixture of bone marrow–derived cells with a scaffold of either collagen powder or hyaluronic acid membrane in 48 subjects. At average 29-month follow-up, the AOFAS score improved from 64 to 91 and histologic analysis showed cartilage remodeling, although not completely hyaline cartilage. Second-look arthroscopies of 5 subjects showed 3 ankles with intact regenerated cartilage layer, whereas 2 had hypertrophic regenerated tissue that was shaved.[58]

A follow-up of these subjects had 41 subjects with 48-month follow-up. The AOFAS scores decreased to a mean of 82. MRIs were obtained for 20 subjects, which showed complete filling in 45%, hypertrophic filling in 45%, and incomplete filling in 10%. The clinical score did correlate with the percent of regenerated tissue. Effusion was evident in only 1 subject (5%), whereas 12 subjects (60%) had subchondral edema.[68]

Hannon and colleagues[71] compared 22 subjects who had bone marrow stimulation with concentrated bone marrow aspirate injected into the lesion with 12 subjects who had bone marrow stimulation alone. For the bone marrow aspirate group, after bone marrow stimulation was performed and bleeding was visualized, 3 mL of concentrated bone marrow aspirate was injected under a dry arthroscope into the defect site. Both groups had significant improvement in preoperative versus postoperative FAOS and SF-12 scores but the improvement between groups was not clinically significant. Postoperative MRI scans showed that the addition of BMAC resulted in improved cartilage border integration and less fissuring and fibrillation.[69]

Kennedy and Murawski[70] harvested OATS from the ipsilateral knee and bathed the graft in 4 mL of BMAC. It was unknown how long the graft was in contact with the BMAC. There were 72 subjects with average 28-month follow-up. FAOS scores improved from 53 to 86 and SF-12 scores improved from 59 to 88. There were 3 donor-site minor complications: 2 resolved from cortisone shot and 1 required knee scope for debridement of scar.[71]

SUMMARY

- OATS is a viable treatment of large OLTs and has low donor-site morbidity.
- Fresh osteochondral talar allograft is also a viable treatment of large OLTs and allows the surgeon to reconstruct difficult geometry of the talus.
- ACI has been shown to have good long-term outcomes but requires multiple procedures.
- Biologics as stand-alone treatment or concomitant procedure for OLT as has promising results in a limited number of studies.

REFERENCES

1. Saxena A, Eakin C. Articular talar injuries in athletes: results of microfracture and autogenous bone graft. Am J Sports Med 2007;35(10): 1680–7.

2. Hintermann B, Regazzoni P, Lampert C, et al. Arthroscopic findings in acute fractures of the ankle. J Bone Joint Surg Br 2000;82-B(3):345–51.

3. Nosewicz TL, Beerekamp MS, De Muinck Keizer RJ, et al. Prospective computed tomographic analysis of osteochondral lesions of the ankle joint associated with ankle fractures. Foot Ankle Int 2016; 37(8):829–34.

4. Regier M, Petersen JP, Hamurcu A, et al. High incidence of osteochondral lesions after open reduction and internal fixation of displaced ankle fractures: Medium-term follow-up of 100 cases. Injury 2016;47(3):757–61.

5. Loomer R, Fischer C, Lloyd-Smith R, et al. Osteochondral lesions of the talus. Am J Sports Med 1993;21(1):13–9.

6. Stroud CC, Marks RM. Imaging of osteochondral lesions of the talus. Foot Ankle Clin 2000;5(1): 119–33.

7. Berndt AL, Harty M. Osteochondritis dissecans of the ankle joint; report of a case simulating a fracture of the talus. J Bone Joint Surg Am 1959; 41-A(4):988–1020.

8. Wodicka R, Ferkel E, Ferkel R. Osteochondral lesions of the ankle. Foot Ankle Int 2016;37(9): 1023–34.

9. Dunlap BJ, Ferkel RD, Applegate GR. The "LIFT" lesion: lateral inverted osteochondral fracture of the talus. Arthroscopy 2013;29(11):1826–33.

10. Choi WJ, Park KK, Kim BS, et al. Osteochondral lesion of the talus: is there a critical defect size for poor outcome? Am J Sports Med 2009;37(10):1974–80.

11. Ramponi L, Yasui Y, Murawski CD, et al. Lesion size is a predictor of clinical outcomes after bone marrow stimulation for osteochondral lesions of the talus: a systematic review. Am J Sports Med 2016. [Epub ahead of print].

12. Choi WJ, Choi GW, Kim JS, et al. Prognostic significance of the containment and location of osteochondral lesions of the talus: independent adverse outcomes associated with uncontained lesions of the talar shoulder. Am J Sports Med 2013;41(1):126–33.

13. Doets HC, van der Plaat LW, Klein JP. Medial malleolar osteotomy for the correction of varus deformity during total ankle arthroplasty: results in 15 ankles. Foot Ankle Int 2008;29(2):171–7.

14. Gobbi A, Francisco RA, Lubowitz JH, et al. Osteochondral lesions of the talus: randomized controlled trial comparing chondroplasty, microfracture, and osteochondral autograft transplantation. Arthroscopy 2006;22(10):1085–92.

15. Sammarco GJ, Makwana NK. Treatment of talar osteochondral lesions using local osteochondral graft. Foot Ankle Int 2002;23(8):693–8.

16. Emre TY, Ege T, Cift HT, et al. Open mosaicplasty in osteochondral lesions of the talus: a prospective study. J Foot Ankle Surg 2012;51(5):556–60.

17. Imhoff AB, Paul J, Ottinger B, et al. Osteochondral transplantation of the talus: long-term clinical and magnetic resonance imaging evaluation. Am J Sports Med 2011;39(7):1487–93.

18. Hu Y, Guo Q, Jiao C, et al. Treatment of large cystic medial osteochondral lesions of the talus with autologous osteoperiosteal cylinder grafts. Arthroscopy 2013;29(8):1372–9.

19. Kim YS, Park EH, Kim YC, et al. Factors associated with the clinical outcomes of the osteochondral autograft transfer system in osteochondral lesions of the talus: second-look arthroscopic evaluation. Am J Sports Med 2012;40(12):2709–19.

20. Hintermann B, Wagener J, Knupp M, et al. Treatment of extended osteochondral lesions of the talus with a free vascularised bone graft from the medial condyle of the femur. Bone Joint J 2015;97-B(9):1242–9.

21. Chen W, Tang K, Yuan C, et al. Intermediate results of large cystic medial osteochondral lesions of the talus treated with osteoperiosteal cylinder autografts from the medial tibia. Arthroscopy 2015;31(8):1557–64.

22. de l'Escalopier N, Barbier O, Mainard D, et al. Outcomes of talar dome osteochondral defect repair using osteocartilaginous autografts: 37 cases of Mosaicplasty. Orthop Traumatol Surg Res 2015;101(1):97–102.

23. Scranton P, McDermott J. Treatment of type V osteochondral lesions of the talus with ipsilateral knee osteochondral autografts. Foot Ankle Int 2001;22(5):380–4.

24. Kreuz PC, Steinwachs M, Erggelet C, et al. Mosaicplasty with autogenous talar autograft for osteochondral lesions of the talus after failed primary arthroscopic management: a prospective study with a 4-year follow-up. Am J Sports Med 2006;34(1):55–63.

25. Lee CH, Chao KH, Huang GS, et al. Osteochondral autografts for osteochondritis dissecans of the talus. Foot Ankle Int 2003;24(11):815–22.

26. Al-Shaikh RA, Chou LB, Mann JA, et al. Autologous osteochondral grafting for talar cartilage defects. Foot Ankle Int 2002;23(5):381–9.

27. Flynn S, Ross KA, Hannon CP, et al. Autologous osteochondral transplantation for osteochondral lesions of the talus. Foot Ankle Int 2016;37(4):363–72.

28. Paul J, Sagstetter A, Kriner M, et al. Donor-site morbidity after osteochondral autologous transplantation for lesions of the talus. J Bone Joint Surg Am 2009;91(7):1683–8.

29. Fraser EJ, Savage-Elliott I, Yasui Y, et al. Clinical and MRI donor site outcomes following autologous osteochondral transplantation for talar osteochondral lesions. Foot Ankle Int 2016;37(9):968–76.

30. Paul J, Sagstetter M, Lämmle L, et al. Sports activity after osteochondral transplantation of the talus. Am J Sports Med 2012;40(4):870–4.

31. Ross AW, Murawski CD, Fraser EJ, et al. Autologous osteochondral transplantation for osteochondral lesions of the talus: does previous bone marrow stimulation negatively affect clinical outcome? Arthroscopy 2016;32(7):1377–83.

32. Bedi A, Feeley BT, William RJ 3rd. Management of articular cartilage defects of the knee [review]. J Bone Joint Surg Am 2010;92(4):994–1009.

33. Enneking WF, Campanacci DA. Retrieved human allografts: a clinicopathological study. J Bone Joint Surg Am 2001;83-A(7):971–86.

34. LaPrade RF, Botker J, Herzog M, et al. Refrigerated osteoarticular allografts to treat articular cartilage defects of the femoral condyles. A Prospective Outcomes Study. J Bone Joint Surg Am 2009;91(4):805–11.

35. Pomajzl RJ, Baker EA, Baker KC, et al. Case series with histopathologic and radiographic analyses following failure of fresh osteochondral allografts of the talus. Foot Ankle Int 2016;37(9):958–67.

36. Gross AE, Agnidis Z, Hutchison CR. Osteochondral defects of the talus treated with fresh osteochondral

allograft transplantation. Foot Ankle Int 2001;22(5): 385–91.

37. Raikin SM. Fresh osteochondral allografts for large-volume cystic osteochondral defects of the talus. J Bone Joint Surg Am 2009;91(12):2818–26.

38. Görtz S, De Young AJ, Bugbee WD. Fresh osteochondral allografting for osteochondral lesions of the talus. Foot Ankle Int 2010;31(4):283–90.

39. Hahn DB, Aanstoos ME, Wilkins RM. Osteochondral lesions of the talus treated with fresh talar allografts. Foot Ankle Int 2010;31(4):277–82.

40. El-Rashidy H, Villacis D, Omar I, et al. Fresh osteochondral allograft for the treatment of cartilage defects of the talus: a retrospective review. J Bone Joint Surg Am 2011;93(17):1634–40.

41. Adams SB Jr, Viens NA, Easley ME, et al. Midterm results of osteochondral lesions of the talar shoulder treated with fresh osteochondral allograft transplantation. J Bone Joint Surg Am 2011;93(7): 648–54.

42. Haene R, Qamirani E, Story RA, et al. Intermediate outcomes of fresh talar osteochondral allografts for treatment of large osteochondral lesions of the talus. J Bone Joint Surg Am 2012;94(12):1105–10.

43. Orr J, Dunn J, Heida K, et al. Results and Functional Outcomes of Structural Fresh Osteochondral Allograft Transfer for Treatment of Osteochondral Lesions of the Talus in a Highly Active Population. Foot Ankle Spec 2017;10(2):125–32.

44. Ahmad J, Jones K. Comparison of osteochondral autografts and allografts for treatment of recurrent or large talar osteochondral lesions. Foot Ankle Int 2016;37:40–50.

45. Zhu Y, Xu X. Osteochondral autograft transfer combined with cancellous allografts for large cystic osteochondral defect of the talus. Foot Ankle Int 2016;37(10):1113–8.

46. Kraeutler MJ, Chahla J, Dean CS, et al. Current concepts review update: osteochondral lesions of the talus. Foot Ankle Int 2017;38(3):331–42.

47. Giannini S, Battaglia M, Buda R, et al. Surgical treatment of osteochondral lesions of the talus by open-field autologous chondrocyte implantation: a 10-year follow-up clinical and magnetic resonance imaging T2-mapping evaluation. Am J Sports Med 2009;37(Suppl 1):112S–8S.

48. Giannini S, Buda R, Vannini F, et al. Arthroscopic autologous chondrocyte implantation in osteochondral lesions of the talus: surgical technique and results. Am J Sports Med 2008;36(5):873–80.

49. Giannini S, Buda R, Ruffilli A, et al. Arthroscopic autologous chondrocyte implantation in the ankle joint. Knee Surg Sports Traumatol Arthrosc 2014; 22(6):1311–9.

50. Lee KT, Choi YS, Lee YK, et al. Comparison of MRI and arthroscopy in modified MOCART scoring system after autologous chondrocyte implantation for osteochondral lesion of the talus. Orthopedics 2011;34(8):e356–62.

51. Nam EK, Ferkel RD, Applegate GR. Autologous chondrocyte implantation of the ankle: a 2- to 5-year follow-up. Am J Sports Med 2009;37(2):274–84.

52. Kwak SK, Kern BS, Ferkel RD, et al. Autologous chondrocyte implantation of the ankle: 2- to 10-year results. Am J Sports Med 2014;42(9): 2156–64.

53. Baums MH, Heidrich G, Schultz W, et al. The surgical technique of autologous chondrocyte transplantation of the talus with use of a periosteal graft. Surgical technique. J Bone Joint Surg Am 2007;89(Suppl 2 Pt 2):170–82.

54. Schneider TE, Karaikudi S. Matrix-Induced Autologous Chondrocyte Implantation (MACI) grafting for osteochondral lesions of the talus. Foot Ankle Int 2009;30(9):810–4.

55. Giza E, Sullivan M, Ocel D, et al. Matrix-induced autologous chondrocyte implantation of talus articular defects. Foot Ankle Int 2010;31(9):747–53.

56. Valderrabano V, Miska M, Leumann A, et al. Reconstruction of osteochondral lesions of the talus with autologous spongiosa grafts and autologous matrix-induced chondrogenesis. Am J Sports Med 2013;41(3):519–27.

57. Wiewiorski M, Werner L, Paul J, et al. Sports activity after reconstruction of osteochondral lesions of the talus with autologous spongiosa grafts and autologous matrix-induced chondrogenesis. Am J Sports Med 2016;44(10):2651–8.

58. Cerrato R. Particulated Juvenile articular cartilage allograft transplantation for osteochondral lesions of the talus. Foot Ankle Clin N Am 2013;18:79–87.

59. Fortier LA, Chapman HS, Pownder SL, et al. Bio-Cartilage improves cartilage repair compared with microfracture alone in an equine model of full-thickness cartilage loss. Am J Sports Med 2016; 44(9):2366–74.

60. Desai S. Surgical treatment of a tibial osteochondral defect with debridement, marrow stimulation, and micronized allograft cartilage matrix: report of an all-arthroscopic technique. J Foot Ankle Surg 2016r;55(2):279–82.

61. Kruse DL, Ng A, Paden M, et al. Arthroscopic De Novo NT juvenile allograft cartilage implantation in the talus: a case presentation. J Foot Ankle Surg 2012;51:218–21.

62. Coetzee JC, Giz E, Schon LC, et al. Treatment of osteochondral lesions of the talus with particulated juvenile cartilage. Foot Ankle Int 2013;34(9): 1205–11.

63. Lanham NS, Carroll JJ, Cooper MT, et al. A comparison of outcomes of particulated juvenile articular cartilage and bone marrow aspirate concentrate for articular cartilage lesions of the talus. Foot Ankle Spec 2016. [Epub ahead of print].

64. Mei-Dan O, Carmont MR, Laver L, et al. Platelet rich plasma or hyaluronate in the management of osteochondral lesions of the talus. Am J Sports Med 2012;40(3):534–41.

65. Gormeli G, Karakaplan M, Gormeli CA, et al. Clinical effects of platelet-rich plasma and hyaluronic acid as an additional therapy for talar osteochondral lesions treated with microfracture surgery: a prospective randomized clinical trial. Foot Ankle Int 2015;36:891–900.

66. Guney A, Akar M, Karaman I, et al. Clinical outcomes of platelet rich plasma (PRP) as an adjunct to microfracture surgery in osteochondral lesions of the talus. Knee Surg Sports Traumatol Arthrosc 2015;23(8):2384–9.

67. Guney A, Yurdakul E, Karaman I, et al. Medium-term outcomes of mosaicplasty versus arthroscopic microfracture with or without platelet-rich plasma in the treatment of osteochondral lesions of the talus. Knee Surg Sports Traumatol Arthrosc 2016; 24(4):1293–8.

68. Giannini S, Buda R, Vannini F, et al. One-step bone marrow derived cell transplantation in talar osteochondral lesions. Clin Orthop Relat Res 2009; 467(12):3307–20.

69. Giannini S, Buda R, Battaglia M, et al. One-step repair in talar osteochondral lesions: 4-year clinical results and t2-mapping capability in outcome prediction. Am J Sports Med 2013; 41(3):511–8.

70. Kennedy JG, Murawski CD. The treatment of osteochondral lesions of the talus with autologous osteochondral transplantation and bone marrow aspirate concentrate: surgical technique. Cartilage 2011;2:327–36.

71. Hannon CP, Ross KA, Murawski CD, et al. Arthroscopic bone marrow stimulation and concentrated bone marrow aspirate for osteochondral lesions of the talus: a case-control study of functional and magnetic resonance observation of cartilage repair tissue outcomes. Arthroscopy 2016;32(2):339–47.

Index

Note: Page numbers of article titles are in **boldface** type.

Orthop Clin N Am 48 (2017) 385–389
http://dx.doi.org/10.1016/S0030-5898(17)30088-3
0030-5898/17

Moving?

Make sure your subscription moves with you!

To notify us of your new address, find your **Clinics Account Number** (located on your mailing label above your name), and contact customer service at:

Email: journalscustomerservice-usa@elsevier.com

800-654-2452 (subscribers in the U.S. & Canada)
314-447-8871 (subscribers outside of the U.S. & Canada)

Fax number: 314-447-8029

Elsevier Health Sciences Division
Subscription Customer Service
3251 Riverport Lane
Maryland Heights, MO 63043

*To ensure uninterrupted delivery of your subscription, please notify us at least 4 weeks in advance of move.

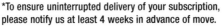

Printed and bound by CPI Group (UK) Ltd, Croydon, CR0 4YY

08/05/2025

01864699-0017